The Secrets of S1

A practical guide to v
to pre

The Secrets of
STOPPING
HAIR LOSS

by

Stella Weller

THORSONS PUBLISHERS LIMITED
Wellingborough, Northamptonshire

First published February 1985
Second Impression May 1985

British Library Cataloguing in Publication Data

Weller, Stella
    The secrets of stopping hair loss.
    1. Baldness
    I. Title
    616.5'46   RL91

    ISBN 0-7225-0942-1

Printed and bound in Great Britain

CONTENTS

INTRODUCTION

Hair loss has unquestionably increased in the last few decades. There is greater incidence of balding, not only among males of all ages, but also among a growing number of females. So remarks Philip Kingsley, a foremost British trichologist (hair scientist). This was foretold by experts, among them American dermatologist (skin specialist) Irwin I. Lubowe. He forecast that by the 1970s, hair loss — partial or total — would be experienced by about 30 per cent more American men than previously. His prophecy, which is equally pertinent to other advanced nations, seems to have come to pass.

Moreover, anthropologists (those specializing in the study of man) have predicted that the next century will see whole nations of bald-pated men. If this happens, the male hirsute head will become a very rare phenomenon indeed!

Hair loss, then, has become a matter of much concern, not only among men, but also among an alarmingly increasing number of women. A leading trichologist, for instance, now treats 25 per cent more women than before in his London and New York clinics for thinning hair. Expert projections indicate that after puberty, about 80 per cent of all men, and about 20 per cent of all women, will experience some degree of hair loss ranging from 'apparent' to 'obvious'.

But anyone who now declares that baldness is incurable must be viewed with suspicion. In fact, Dr Lubowe has asserted that the pessimistic prophecies of the hairless man of the future may now be more critically assessed than heretofore. Such predictions are not based on long-term trends. They have not made allowance for scientific progress. And *progress has been made.* Even physicians who, in times past, insisted that baldness was impossible to cure, are now changing their attitude in the light of new findings. As one expert notes, baldness is not always inevitable, and the amount and rate of hair loss can often be diminished with correct treatment; the branch of medicine dealing with the hair and scalp and skin (dermatology) has made too many significant advances for progressive hair loss to be the puzzle it once was. So, too, have other specialities, including anthropology and biology (the science of life and living things). And now, more than ever before, causes of 'permanent' baldness are being demonstrated as instances of temporary hair loss only. For hair follicles (the sheaths in which hairs grow) can remain alive for up to a quarter of a century of seeming inactivity, and as long as they hold even the slightest potential for renewed activity, *there is hope.*

This book examines factors influencing hair loss and suggests practical ways of dealing with them. It provides aids to help combat those influences that would decimate the hairs on your head. It offers new hope for renewed hair growth. As you read on, you will discover various aspects of that hope — secrets of stopping hair loss and encouraging hair growth. These, used in combination, will produce the best results, because mounting evidence convincingly indicates that baldness is not due to any one cause, but to *a combination of causes.*

There are no instant cures, though. You must be patient. The growth period for hair is between two and six years, and for about three months there is a rest period (the telogen phase) in the normal cycle of hair growth in which about 10 per cent of scalp hair ceases to grow and prepares for shedding. It takes a year to grow about six inches of it. Often when hair is being shed, the hair follicles beneath the thinning section of scalp are in the resting phase.

But many of us are, unfortunately, in too much of a hurry nowadays. Understandably, those experiencing what appears to be advancing hair loss are in even more of a hurry. They are prime targets for well-meaning (and not-so-well-meaning) hair salons and clinics that make extravagant claims and offer enticements that are often emotionally and financially costly as well as unsatisfactory or disappointing in the long term.

Please do not panic if you do not see immediate results. Persevere. Your rewards will be proportionate to your conscientiousness, your persistence and your patience. Good luck!

1.

HAIR LOSS: TYPES AND CAUSES

Every day you and I lose between twenty and sixty hairs. This is normal hair loss. It is only when the loss of hair exceeds its rate of new growth that thinning becomes noticeable. It is only when you lose nearly 40 per cent of your natural head covering does its disappearance become evident enough to be regarded as abnormal hair loss or incipient baldness.

The medical word for abnormal hair loss is *alopecia* (pronounced 'al-o-pee-she-ah'), and comes from the Greek word 'alopekia', which bears the unattractive meaning of 'fox mange'. It denotes a natural or abnormal baldness, or deficiency of hair, partial or complete, localized or generalized.

Here is an impressive list of the types of alopecia, and what each signifies ('A' is used as an abbreviation for 'alopecia').

A. adnata	congenital baldness or baldness at birth
A. areata	well-defined patches of baldness that leave the scalp smooth and white; patchy baldness
A. congenital	baldness due to the absence of hair bulbs at birth
A. follicularis	hair loss due to the inflammation of the hair follicles
A. furfuracea	chronic hair loss marked by dandruff and itching
A. neurotica	baldness following a nervous disease or injury to the nervous system
A. pityroides	loss of both scalp and body hair with excessive shedding of skin cells, reminiscent of bran flakes
A. prematura	early or premature baldness

A. senilis	baldness of old age
A. simplex	premature baldness
A. symptomatica	hair loss following prolonged fevers during the course of a disease, or from changes in internal secretions
A. totalis	loss of hair from the entire scalp
A. toxica	loss of hair, thought to be due to the toxins of infectious disease
A. universalis	general loss of hair from all parts of the body

Causes of hair loss — general

The explanations opposite the types of hair loss just given will give clues as to the causes. These fall, roughly, into the following categories:

- Hereditary factors
- The ageing process
- Illnesses and infectious diseases
- Hormonal imbalance
- Nervous disorders and nervous system injury
- Toxic substances (drugs, for example)
- Injury and impairment

Early and old-age baldness (A. prematura and A. senilis, respectively) are so similar in appearance that they have come to be known as 'pattern baldness', or 'common baldness' which, as the latter term signifies, is the most common type of baldness.

Pattern or common baldness

Responsible researchers have estimated that more than 90 per cent of all causes of abnormal hair loss are in the pattern-type category.

Characteristically, the hairline starts to recede, or hair loss becomes noticeable at the crown of the head and progresses toward the forehead. Irrespective of where this hair loss begins, it denudes much of the scalp as it continues, leaving only a fringe reminiscent of a horseshoe. It is a pattern with which we are all becoming increasingly familiar.

Causes of pattern or common baldness

Apart from heredity factors, all causes contributing to this most common form of hair loss fall into these categories:

- Seborrhoea (excessive dandruff)
- Scalp infections
- General ill-health or disease
- Scalp injury
- Impaired blood circulation
- Hormonal imbalance
- Nutritional inadequacy or deficiency.

Seborrhoea (dandruff)

Seborrhoea is a functional disease of the sebaceous (oil-secreting) glands of the skin which, of course, includes the scalp. These glands are located in the second layer of scalp tissue and are usually linked to the hair follicle. They secrete an oily substance called *sebum*, which helps to keep the hair resilient.

Seborrhoea is characterized by an increase in the amount, and sometimes by an alteration in the quality, of sebum. The production of sebum is influenced by diet, metabolism (the building-up and breaking-down of tissue cells), emotional factors, endocrine (internal secreting) glandular function, and by the blood circulation.

There are various types of seborrhoea (subsequently represented by the abbreviation 'S.'), but the one that concerns us here is *S. capiti,* or seborrhoea of the scalp, of which *S. sicca* (*sicca* meaning 'dry'), popularly called dandruff, is the most common.

Dandruff appears on the scalp and behind and in the ears as small, whitish crusts or scales.

Causes of dandruff
Excessive dandruff has been linked to hormonal imbalance by experts on baldness, including an authority on the subject, Dr J. B. Hamilton.

If this condition is allowed to persist untreated, the nutrition of the hair is interfered with and a balding process sets in.

S. sicca, the most common form of dandruff, is a prime

suspect in the insidious process of abnormal hair loss. The bulk of available evidence suggests that it is caused by chemical reactions occurring inside the body, and that this reaction is associated with stress, faulty diet and the indiscriminate use of hair cosmetics.

Treating dandruff
The first prerequisite of the effective treatment of dandruff is, of course, to determine its cause. You may need to consult your physician, who may in turn refer you to a dermatologist to help get to the root of the matter. Certainly, if the condition persists, this is the route you should take.

Meantime, there are several aspects of strategic attack on dandruff to observe. One is *scrupulous hair hygiene* (see Chapter 12). Another is diet modification: restrict carbohydrate (sugar and starch) intake; cut down on the consumption of saturated fats (mainly of animal origin); avoid the addition of salt to food, both when cooking it and at the table. (Please read Chapter 7 for helpful guidelines. The diet suggested will do a great deal to help to counteract the overactivity of the sebaceous glands.)

Yet another aspect of anti-dandruff strategy is restoring harmony to the endocrine glandular system. Experts suspect that an increase in androgens (male hormones) contributes to seborrhoea. You will find the gland exercises in Chapter 9 useful in stimulating the endocrine glands to promote normality of function.

Knowledgeable researchers remark that skin conditions, like seborrhoea, are affected by the emotions. This will not surprise you when you learn to appreciate the intimate link between the nervous system and every other body system. There are nerve endings all over the body, no less so in the scalp. Anxiety and other forms of nervous tension over-stimulate these nerve endings, which in turn influence the structures they supply to produce a sort of empathic response. These structures are then likely to overreact (and they often do) and overproduce, as happens in seborrhoea. The result, in a nutshell, is that the balance of the entire human organism is upset. The body's natural defence mechanism weakens. Infection finds a ready breeding ground.

Do practise, every day, some of the stress-reducing techniques given in Chapter 10 to help you to meet emotional challenges with a greater degree of composure than you may now be able to do.

Local applications
Drugstores and chemists sell the whole gamut of anti-dandruff treatments and shampoos. Many of them are medicated or contain ingredients that, in the long term, may be potentially harmful to the body. Many of them make extravagant claims. All are stopgap measures, and *none can be relied upon* to clear up what can sometimes be a stubborn condition.

Herbal and other natural anti-dandruff remedies

Herbs
The following herbs are proven remedies to counteract dandruff:

- Burdock
- Nettle
- Rosemary
- Sage
- Willow
- Yarrow

These anti-dandruff remedies have been used for decades (some for centuries) in the successful treatment of dandruff. They have proven effective in halting hair loss resulting from persisting dandruff, in strengthening the hair and in helping to revitalize hair growth.

How to make them
Brew a 'tea' of your selected herb or herbs by infusing one tablespoon of herb(s) in a pint of boiling water. Leave the infusion for half an hour. Cool and strain it. Store it in a clean jar or bottle and use some of it daily, if possible.

How to use
You may use your herbal preparation either as a pre-shampoo, anti-dandruff hair conditioner, as a post-shampoo rinse, or as part of your daily manual scalp massage routine.
    For the former, pour some of the liquid into a shallow

container. Dip all your fingers into it periodically as you carry out the manual massage described in Chapter 13.

Leave the application on the hair and scalp for ten minutes while you lie down and relax (see also Chapter 13), or otherwise occupy yourself. Then shampoo your hair as directed in Chapter 12.

As a rinse, use your herbal 'tea' after shampooing your hair, to help to remove all traces of shampoo and any remaining flecks of foreign matter.

If you add to your herbal infusion a level tablespoonful of boric acid (available from chemists and drug stores), which has mild antiseptic properties, it will enhance the effectiveness of the herbal treatment. Be sure to mix the two ingredients together thoroughly before applying the solution to the scalp as previously directed.

Boric acid is a very old remedy for dandruff. You may use it on its own, moistened with a little water. Rub it well into the scalp (being careful not to tug at the hair), then rinse it out well with warm water. You can carry out this procedure before your routine shampoo.

Yogurt
Rub half a cupful of plain, unsweetened yogurt and massage it, a little at a time, into the scalp.

Drape a towel around your head, or put on a bathcap or other head-covering and leave the yogurt to do its work for one hour. This is an excellent time to make use of your slant board — lie on it up to twenty minutes to treat the scalp to a surge of fresh blood that will enhance the removal of impurities from that area.

An hour after the yogurt application, thoroughly rinse the hair with warm water. You may then shampoo your hair.

Yogurt, of course, is good to eat, too. Health experts say that it benefits the natural flora of the intestines — the friendly bacteria that help to synthesize the B vitamins, which are essential for healthy hair growth and reinvigoration.

Other causes of common baldness

As we age, fewer hairs re-enter the growth cycle, so there tends to be a general thinning of scalp hair. This is usually more apparent in men than in women. But not always, especially nowadays, when there appears to be a sharp rise of hair loss among career women. In relatively undeveloped countries like parts of Africa, India, and Mexico, however, people retain generous hair growth to a ripe old age.

Scalp infections

The most common signs and symptoms of scalp infection are persistent itching, the formation of flakes and crusts, sensitivity of the scalp and hair loss.

Fungus infections like ringworm cause scaly, bald patches on the head. The hair in affected areas breaks off just above scalp level, leaving well-marked stumps. The affected hairs show a characteristic green fluorescence when examined in a darkroom under a special light.

In some cases of ringworm, suppuration occurs: the portions of scalp affected become swollen and inflamed, and exude purulent matter. Ringworm of the scalp is best treated by a doctor or a dermatologist.

General ill-health or disease

Any ailment or disease is potentially harmful to the health of the hair. Hair reflects the nutritional status of its owner, and many nutrition-conscious doctors are now analysing hair samples from their patients for clues as to nutritional inadequacy or deficiency. This is because of the amazing capacity of the hair to reflect in its cells the general health of the body, and thus help in the diagnosis of disease.

In certain diseases (for example, of the thyroid gland), hair loss may be severe enough to generate anxiety, while the anxiety will aggravate the ill-health — a vicious circle.

Removal of the causative factor is, in many cases, the province of a competent physician. If an inadequate diet is suspect, Chapters 4, 5 and 7 will provide much information to help to raise your nutrition level.

If you do not have a daily bowel evacuation, then do please study Chapter 11 and apply the principles given.

Scalp injury

Injury to the scalp can occur in many ways, ranging from burns to the effects of prolonged traction on the hair from a tight perm, hair curlers, tight plaits, ponytails or buns.

Anything that damages the scalp's subsurface tissues, wherein lies the hair's manufacturing plant, can contribute to hair loss. Anything that increases scalp tension or otherwise restricts free blood flow to the hair cells will impair hair growth and regeneration.

Serious injury, such as a burn, requires treatment by a doctor. Lesser injuries, such as those resulting from indiscriminate manipulation of the hair, demand discontinuation of these practices.

Impaired blood circulation

Factors influencing free flow of blood to the hair include tight headwear and head gear, scalp and facial tension, undue tension of the whole body, atherosclerosis (narrowing of blood vessels by fatty deposits within them), and smoking, which particularly restricts the peripheral circulation (at the extremities of the body).

Where a medical condition has been diagnosed, the treatment will of course be prescribed by the doctor. But if your diet is too high in animal fats (from meats and butter, for example), do read Chapter 7 for ways to reduce your intake of these food items. In the same chapter, you will find pointers to help you effectively cut down your consumption of refined sugar and salt, and to increase dietary fibre.

If you are prone to be over-tense, resolve to incorporate into your daily living some of the stress-relieving aids outlined in Chapter 10. And if you are a heavy smoker, it is definitely time to cut down on, or cut out, the tobacco habit.

Hormonal imbalance

Any condition affecting the endocrine glands can affect hair growth and renewal. In particular, disorders of the thyroid gland, located in the neck, are known to promote hair loss. The thyroid gland influences the body's metabolism, and its underactivity, for example, could lead to thinning of the hair.

Other factors influencing hormonal balance include the use of the Pill, and pregnancy.

I recall vividly when the oral contraceptive pill was first being introduced. I was nursing in London and working closely with a gynaecologist/researcher. I shall never forget how thoroughly he screened every young woman who consulted him on contraception, the innumerable questions he asked on medical and family history and on medications being used. I remember, too, the various tests to which he subjected his clients. He referred to those women with healthy oestrogen (female sex hormone) levels as 'oestrogenic young ladies'.

I was appalled, years later, at how readily doctors dispensed the Pill to their clients, without even bothering to find out whether or not the particular pill prescribed would be the one most suitable for the specific person. Abnormal hair loss, although distressing, is the least serious side-effect of such indiscriminate prescription, as the years have shown. We know now that blood clots and other potentially life-threatening conditions can arise from habitual use of such contraceptives.

Birth control pills affect a woman's metabolizing of vitamins and this often leads to anaemia ('iron-poor blood'). It is estimated that about six million persons in Britain and about twenty million in the United States suffer from some form of anaemia.

Women taking birth control pills may need to supplement their diet with certain minerals and vitamins to help to prevent anaemia, which is definitely hazardous to the health of the hair. The Pill, which is a combination of female and male hormones, alters the body's natural hormonal balance. Anything that does this will, without any doubt, affect the health of the hair.

In pregnancy, many hormonal changes take place in the body, often persisting until many weeks after the baby is born. They can produce a sufficient degree of endocrine gland imbalance to effect a frightening loss of scalp hair. This loss, however, is only temporary. Within months of the baby's arrival — earlier perhaps — hair growth resumes its normal pattern. Simply persist in carrying out a scrupulous hair hygiene regimen; remember, too, to avoid any hairdo that pulls unnecessarily on the hair (such as a ponytail or a tight perm).

Nervous disorders and nervous system injury

When we were still in the embryonic stages of life (in the womb), our hair, nails, skin, nervous system and some endocrine glands were all part of the same tissue (the ectoderm). Is it any wonder, then, that certain nervous disorders affect the skin, hair and scalp?

Our emotions are very much under the influence of our endocrine glands (see p. 63). Some even say that we are a product of these glands, which are intimately linked with the nervous system. The nervous system, in turn, is closely connected with the skin through myriad nerve endings. It is therefore not difficult to appreciate that any disorder upsetting this harmonious interrelationship, or any injury to the nervous system (such as a severe burn), could cause abnormal hair loss.

Toxic substances

Several medications or 'drugs', used for long enough or in high doses can cause abnormal hair loss. Among these are antithyroid and anticancer drugs, arsenic preparations, thallium, preparations containing a high proportion of sex hormones, amphetamines and anticoagulants.

It is a wise precaution to familiarize yourself with the possible side-effects of any medication prescribed for you. And if you are taking several medications simultaneously, be aware of the possible effects of their interaction. Ask your doctor or pharmacist for this information. If you are not satisfied with what you are told, or if what you want to know is not forthcoming, local librarians are usually delighted to suggest a good reference work.

Injury and impairment

Anything that contributes to increased tension in the facial and scalp muscles can be considered a contributory factor in hair loss. Anything that restricts the flow of blood to the hair is counterproductive to healthy hair growth and revivication. These include any head injury that leaves much scar tissue, any surgery that produces the same results (including those 'non-scarring' hair-replacement techniques that are being flaunted nowadays — I have yet to see a surgical procedure that does *not* leave a scar!), and tight hair curlers or perms, which can produce a sort of 'traction baldness'.

2.

THE ROOT OF THE MATTER

You know that you are losing hair. You see it in your comb and brush. You notice it on your pillow and in your washbasin. You observe it on your clothing and on the floor. But is it increasing in quantity from day to day, from week to week?

Here is a weekly test you can perform, before shampooing your hair, to help you to determine if your hair loss is advancing. You will need a white towel, a comb and a note placed where you can see it to remind you to do the test each week, preferably on the same day.

The comb test

1. Spread the towel on a table, a counter or on the bed.
2. Lean over the towel.
3. Comb through the hair:
   fifty downstrokes on the right side of the scalp;
   fifty downstrokes on the left side of the scalp;
   fifty downstrokes in the centre of the scalp.
4. Carefully count every hair on the towel and in the comb. Make a note of it on your calendar, or in a notebook kept specifically for this purpose.
5. Clean the towel and keep it handy for next week's test.
6. Repeat this procedure every week, on the same day if possible.

Interpreting the results
If there is no spectacular increase in the hair fall from week to week, you need not be alarmed. Remember, it is the increase in the *rate of fall* and the *persistence* of this increased loss that are significant.

If, however, the twenty-five hairs lost last week increase to thirty-five this week, to forty-five next week, and so on, you must promptly initiate a programme to halt this acceleration of hair loss.

Sometimes, even if there are a hundred hairs in your washbasin, this may represent only a natural turnover, that is, the hair in the basin will be replaced by the same number, and with the same quality of hair, according to the natural hair growth cycle. Periods of increased mental stress, the use of certain medications (such as antithyroid pills and oral contraceptives), or pregnancy, can result in this stepped-up hair loss. With abatement or discontinuation of the causative factors, the usual hair growth pattern generally resumes.

The looking-glass test

Another way of monitoring the extent of your hair loss is to carry out a weekly looking-glass test.

A three-way mirror is the best one to use, but any looking-glass will do. You scrutinize your scalp each week to see if your hair is growing sparser, and keep a record, if you like, of any observations you think relevant or significant.

Meanwhile, here is what you can do to approach and to deal with your problem (imagined or real) in the most intelligent way.

1. Read through Chapter 3 carefully, to gain an appreciation of the structure and function of the scalp and the composition of hair.
2. Read Chapter 1 again, to try to determine what may be some of the contributing causes of *your* hair loss. If you have even the slightest doubt as to what might be precipitating or aggravating your condition, do not hesitate to get help from a physician or a hair or skin specialist.
3. Honestly answer the following questions:

    ● Do you shampoo your hair
      regularly?   Yes _____ No _____
    ● Do you use the right technique?
      (See Chapter 12 for the right
      way)   Yes _____ No _____

- Do you keep your comb and brush scrupulously clean?   Yes _____ No _____
- Do you massage your scalp daily?   Yes _____ No _____
  More than once a day?   Yes _____ No _____
- Is your diet adequate to support healthy hair growth and hair regeneration? (Refer to Chapters 4, 5 and 7 to make sure)   Yes _____ No _____
- Do you have a thorough bowel evacuation at least once a day?   Yes _____ No _____
- Are you inclined to be overtense?   Yes _____ No _____
- Do you practise some form of stress control every day?   Yes _____ No _____
- Do you have a daily exercise regimen?   Yes _____ No _____
- Does your exercise routine include outdoor, aerobic type exercise (such as brisk walking, bicycling, swimming) to stimulate heart and lungs?   Yes _____ No _____
- Does your exercise programme include inverted ('upside-down') or semi-inverted positions?   Yes _____ No _____
- Have you sought medical aid for any skin or scalp disorder, however seemingly unimportant?   Yes _____ No _____
- Have you had a medical checkup within the past year to rule out conditions such as anaemia, high blood pressure, high blood cholesterol level, thyroid disorder, etc.?   Yes _____ No _____
- Are you regularly using barbiturates to help you to sleep?   Yes _____ No _____
- Are you regularly using medications that may aggravate hair loss (such as

antithyroid preparations, oral
contraceptives, etc.)?   Yes ___ No ___

● Do you know the possible side-
effects of medication you are
taking?   Yes ___ No ___

Interpreting the answers

There is no good, bad or indifferent score for the above
questionnaire, which has been formulated to give you insight
into the factors influencing hair growth and renewal. Your
answers will indicate areas of neglect and, I hope, lead you
to rectify shortcomings in your present hair care strategy.

If your hair loss is progressive

After answering the questions in the foregoing questionnaire
and discovering areas of neglect, and after persisting in your
weekly tests and realizing that your hair loss may be
progressing, you may wish — and wisely so — to consult your
doctor. He, in turn, may decide to refer you to a dermatologist.

It is important that you have a good rapport with your
doctor, and that he is sympathetic to your condition and its
associated anxieties.

If he is in a rush, if he does not answer your questions fully,
if he tells you that your problem is 'psychosomatic', if he is
quick to dispense medication without first carefully examining
you and ordering tests, then maybe you are not seeing the
right doctor.

To help you find a suitable doctor, you might like to read
How to Choose and Use Your Doctor by Marvin S. Belsky and
Leonard Gross.

Tests that may be ordered

After careful history-taking and thorough physical
examination, a competent doctor may decide to order specific
tests to rule out (or confirm) the presence of disease that may
be contributing to your hair loss.

Examples of such diseases are liver and thyroid disorders,
anaemia, diabetes, heart disease and ovarian abnormality.

3.
GETTING TO KNOW
YOUR SCALP AND HAIR

In any relationship, the better the partners get to know one another, the better they are able to contribute to each other's growth and wellbeing. The more each party understands the other, the more he or she can help the common cause when things go wrong.

It is no less true that the better you understand the structure and function of your hair and scalp and related structures, the more intelligently you can set about preserving and maintaining their health.

Some readers may feel that this chapter does not concern them. But I do urge you, in the interest of keeping your hair and keeping it healthy, to take the time to at least read it once from beginning to end. Even if you do not retain all the facts, a careful first reading will acquaint you with the workings of structures that have a bearing on your hair growth and give you needed insight into the reasons for the suggestions which follow later in the book.

What is hair?

The other day, as I looked through an old anatomy textbook which I used in my student-nurse days, I came across this sentence: 'The hairs and nails and sebaceous glands are looked upon as appendages of the skin'. And yet, hair is not merely an appendage; it is not simply attached or affixed to the skin (which includes the scalp, of course).

Hair is a living, integral part of your body, just as the heart is. It thrives when the body is healthy; when the body sickens, it empathizes by weakening. In fact, many doctors find clues to what is taking place in the body by looking at the hair, for it is an index to the inner person.

Hair, then, is like a true friend which, as one poet wrote:

Thus, of every grief in heart,
He with thee will bear a part.

Hair is part of the skin, and scalp hair is part of the scalp.

The scalp

According to my medical dictionary, scalp is 'the hairy integument of the head', 'integument' being a biological term for 'covering'.

Scalp includes skin, dense subcutaneous (below the skin) tissue, occipito-frontalis muscle with the galea aponeurotica (which will be explained below), subaponeurotic tissue and the cranial periosteum.

Periosteum
This is a fibrous membrane covering bone; cranial periosteum covers the skull or cranium. It serves as a supporting structure for blood vessels and tendons. It gives protection to the bone and helps in its repair after injury.

Skin
Skin is made up of two parts: an inner layer or *dermis* (true skin), and an outer layer or *epidermis* (false skin). Hair is an extension — an outgrowth, if you like — of the outer layer.

Composition of the epidermis
The epidermis — the outer part of the skin — is composed of tissue known as *stratified epithelium*, that is, it is made up of more than one stratum or horizontal layer of cells.

The outermost layer — nearest the surface — is the *horny layer* of the skin. Its cells are flattened and resemble scales.

The middle layer of cells are called 'prickly cells' because they are interconnected by fine tendrils that give them a prickly appearance when seen through a microscope.

The deepest or basal layer contains columnar-type cells. (Columnar cells line most of the tubes and organs of the body, especially where there is much activity.) This is the *germinate layer* in which cells multiply by *karyokinesis:*they push those above them nearer the surface until the superficial ones are shed.

The lower surface of the epidermis contains depressions into which fit projections on the upper surface of the dermis. This arrangement makes for less damage to the skin, and for a larger area to accommodate nerves and blood vessels.

Composition of the dermis
Because the dermis contains structures that are essential to the health and life of the hair, it is worthy of scrutiny.

It is composed of fibrous tissue, the lower layer of which contains fat cells. It contains nerves, blood vessels, sweat and sebaceous glands and hair follicles. And regardless of the seeming smoothness of any scalp, it has countless tiny openings: pores for the excretion of the sweat glands; follicles or depressions for the hair shafts, and openings of the oil-secreting or sebaceous glands (Figure 1).

The papillae
Beneath each hair shaft is a papilla (Latin for 'nipple', plural: 'papillae'), which resembles a pimple, and which is in fact *the hair's manufacturing plant*. The base of each hair widens and fits snugly into the projection of the papilla.

The papilla contains capillaries (tiny blood vessels) through which the hair receives its nourishment from the body's circulatory system.

Should you pluck out a healthy hair, the papilla will not necessarily be damaged. It will, in due course, manufacture a new hair that will emerge through the follicle. Because the papilla is integrated into the skin tissues, you cannot 'root' it up as you would a plant. What people (some doctors included) call the hair 'root' is the whitish bulb at the base of a jerked-out hair. The papilla is the closest thing to a root that a hair has.

The sebaceous glands
These are located in the dermis or inner layer of skin. Usually, they are linked to the hair follicles, also situated in this layer. They produce a fatty secretion known as *sebum* (see p. 11) which helps to keep the hair supple.

Several factors influence the production of sebum. Among these are the blood circulation, diet, emotional disturbances, endocrine gland stimulation, and metabolism.

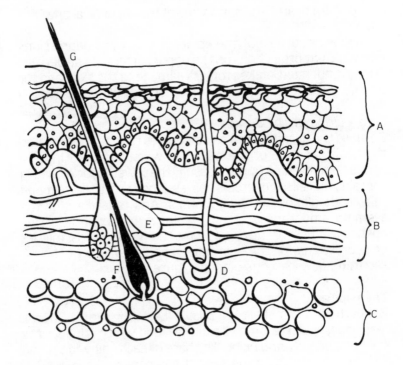

A — Layers of the epidermis
B — Dermis
C — Subcutaneous tissues
D — Sweat gland
E — Sebaceous gland
F — Hair follicle
G — Hair

Figure 1   Cross-section of the human scalp

The functioning of the sebaceous glands seems to have a bearing on the health of the hair and scalp. Overactivity can cause excessive secretion of oil, which in turn may promote or aggravate dandruff. Overactivity, too, is suspected as a factor in an oversupply of androgens (male hormones), which have been linked to common baldness.

Muscles, nerves and blood
We have already looked at the structures of the skin and

underlying tissues. Let us now consider musculature and nerve and blood supply.

The occipito-frontalis muscle

The occipito-frontalis muscle, sometimes referred to simply as the frontalis, runs from the back of the head, over it, to the eyebrows. This muscle includes an intervening *aponeurosis*, which is a flattened, tendon-like structure having the same function as a tendon (a white, glistening, inelastic fibrous band that binds muscle to bone).

The significance of this aponeurosis, which is called the *galea* (Latin for 'helmet'), will become apparent later.

When contracted, the occipito-frontalis muscle raises the eyebrows, wrinkling the forehead horizontally. It also draws the scalp forward.

The nerve supply to this muscle is through the seventh (VIIth) cranial or facial nerve which permits versatility of facial expression, and which has branches that activate the ears.

The blood supply is through the external carotid artery, a branch of one of the body's chief blood vessels. This artery has three branches: the *facial artery*, supplying the lower face; the *temporal artery*, supplying the side of the head near the temples, and the *occipital artery*, which passes to the back of the head, dividing into smaller branches to service this area.

The temporal muscles

The temporal muscles are triangular-shaped muscles at the sides of the head, which raise the lower jaw.

The trigeminal (three-headed) or fifth (Vth) cranial nerve, which also supplies the face, head, and muscles involved with chewing, represents this muscle's nerve supply. The external carotid artery provides its blood supply.

Although not part of the scalp musculature, the following two muscles may have a bearing on the health of the hair and scalp, as will be seen later.

The zygomaticus major and risorius

The zygomaticus major, which draws the angles of the mouth upward, and the risorius, which draws the angles of the mouth outward are muscles of facial expression. If habitually contracted because of tension, say some researchers, they can constrict the blood vessels supplying the scalp, thus impairing nourishment to the hair.

Composition of hair

Let us start at the bottom. From the papilla, a single human hair emerges and tapers upward from its bulb (Figure 2). If your hair is straight, its circumference will be round when seen through a microscope. If it is wavy, it will appear oval. If decidedly curly, it will look flat-sided.

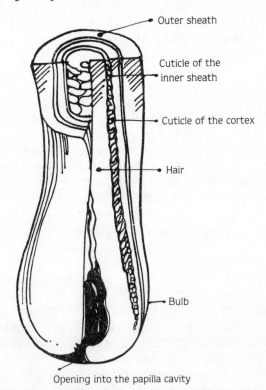

Outer sheath

Cuticle of the inner sheath

Cuticle of the cortex

Hair

Bulb

Opening into the papilla cavity

Figure 2 Structure of the human hair

Mitotic cells
The bulb of the hair follicle is divided into two parts: a lower part, composed of mitotic (or dividing) cells known as undifferentiated cells; an upper part containing differentiated cells that are responsible for producing the inner hair sheath and the hair shaft itself.

Despite phrases like missing something 'by a hair' or a 'hair's breadth', a strand of hair is actually thick enough to be composed of three layers, not unlike the layers of stratified epithelium, described earlier (p. 24).

Hair layers

The outermost or horny layer is known also as the *cuticle* because it is a sturdy, hardened layer of the hair shaft.

The *cortex* or middle layer is composed of elastic material that gives the hair its resilience and flexibility. This is the layer that contains the colouring matter which determines whether you are blond(e), redhead or brunet(te).

The innermost layer or *medulla* is analogous to the marrow of a bone, and it is through it that the hair absorbs its nourishment.

Of great significance, especially to those concerned with preserving as much scalp hair as possible, is the fact that the molecules of each layer of hair are laced together in seven coiled strands. Scientists now believe that these strands are held together and prevented from unravelling by a constant supply of protein. Thus any practice that has the potential to destroy this protein bond is, of course, a threat to the life of the hair.

Hair muscles

It is no fallacy that on occasion, such as when you are frightened, your hair literally stands on end. Attached to the hair shafts are tiny muscles called the *arrectores pilorum*, or erector pili muscles which, as the name suggests, cause the hairs to be erect.

Under the influence of nervous excitation, these muscles contract and cause the hairs to which they are linked to become rigid. Similarly, when you are cold the goose-pimples you may experience are the result of the action of the arrectores pilorum.

Thus, the hair is affected by the state of the nervous system and by the condition of the circulatory system. As such, it is very much interrelated to the functioning of the entire human organism: body, mind and emotions. When you ponder on the opulence of the nerve and blood supply to the head, you will have no difficulty appreciating that whatever adversely affects them will, in the long term, be to the detriment of the hair with which they are inextricably bound up.

Function of the hair

Recently, I read a book on hair transplants, in which the author declared that hair served no purpose but that of adornment.

No one will dispute that a luxuriant head of hair is a desirable personal embellishment or that it can be an asset (indeed, it is a secondary sexual characteristic). But hair has functions other than enhancing appearance or self-image. Hair is the body's chief protector from external damage: it acts as a solar screen and as a valuable sensory structure. Scalp hair helps to keep the head warm and protect the skull from minor injuries.

The hairs on your head are numbered

Researchers and students of dermatology (the science of the skin) agree that anyone endowed with a good head of hair will have between 90 000 and 140 000 hairs, with natural blond(e)s close to the top figure, redheads near the bottom, and brunet(te)s somewhere near the 108 000 mark.

Hair growth cycle

Healthy scalp hair grows at an average daily rate of approximately 0.35mm (1/72 inch), that is, about 2.5cm (1 inch) every 2½ months.

Hair has a long growth period (the *anagen* stage), which normally lasts between two and six years, and a short rest period (the *telogen* stage) of about three months' duration.

At any one time, about 85 per cent of scalp hair is in the growing phase, and about 15 per cent is in the resting stage. It is in this latter stage that hair is gradually being shed. The hair you find in your comb and brush and washbasin, as well as on your pillow, is likely to be in the resting stage and ready to be shed. This gives healthy papillae a chance to manufacture new hairs.

In between the active hair growing and the resting or quiescent phases, there's a period of transition known as the *catagen* stage.

Of interest is an observation made years ago by Dr Chase, a Brown University biologist, while studying hair growth. Dr Chase noted that if the hair of an animal was plucked while in the resting (telogen) stage, the active (anagen) phase was somehow induced, and came about more quickly than it would otherwise have done.

The implications of this finding remind me of an incident that took place in my own home not long ago.

One of our dragon plants — a cluster of three shoots — began to droop, unlike its companion which we bought at the same plant shop. We followed to the letter all the instructions for its care — exposure to light, watering, trimming of leaves, etc. — but to no avail. The plant continued to languish until one of the shoots finally withered and died. As if in sympathy, the two remaining shoots went on a sort of hunger strike. They began to wilt, lost leaves and all but followed their deceased companion into extinction.

One day, as carefully as I could, I eased the dead shoot from its container. It yielded more easily than I had expected. From that day on, there was no mistake — the two other shoots gradually showed signs of strengthening until, today, they stand proud and vigorous and healthy looking. The change was indeed dramatic.

It seemed that the ailing shoot, doomed to die, was sapping the life force from its neighbours in seeming desperation to survive. Once removed, however, it allowed the others more room to breathe, as it were, and to absorb needed nutrients of which they were formerly being robbed.

Is it not conceivable, then, that hair about to be shed diminishes the nourishment available to the healthy hair, and that the sooner one is rid of it the better for the wellbeing of the hair in the active growing phase? For this reason, the advice of one expert is in order: with courage and brush in hand, do not hesitate to clear away debris in the form of hairs that are ready for removal anyway. (I want to add, though, that brushing should definitely not be done with a vengeance!)

Normal hair loss
The normal daily rate of shedding is estimated between twenty and sixty hairs. Some authorities say that it may be as many as 100 hairs. As one gets older, the rate of loss exceeds the rate of growth of new hair; but only when you are bereft of about 40 per cent of your hair does thinning become obvious.

4.

WONDER FOODS FOR YOUR HAIR

Before taking a look at individual nutrients needed for healthy hair — what they are, what their functions are and what are their best food sources — it is relevant and of value to know how the hair is fed. In this chapter I shall outline how the food you take into your body passes into the bloodstream which feeds every part of your body, from head to toes.

After food has been eaten, its digestion — which begins in the mouth — continues in the stomach and small intestine. Nearly all the absorption of digested food takes place in the small intestine.

Blood circulation

The blood that has circulated through the stomach and intestine is collected by the *portal vein* (veins are blood vessels that carry blood *to* the heart) and taken to the liver. Here, it breaks up into smaller blood vessels which unite with similar ones, joining the *hepatic artery* (arteries carry blood *from* the heart) (Figure 3).

This dual blood supply is then collected by a system of veins, which eventually convey blood from the liver to the *inferior vena cava* (the principal vein draining the lower portion of the body). The inferior vena cava enters the upper *right* chamber *(atrium)* of the heart, whence it proceeds into the lower right chamber *(ventricle)*.

When the ventricle contracts, it pumps the blood into the *pulmonary* (lung) artery which divides and takes the blood to both lungs. In the lungs, the blood gives up its impurities, gathered in the tissues, and receives oxygen in exchange.

From here, the blood is carried back to the heart by way

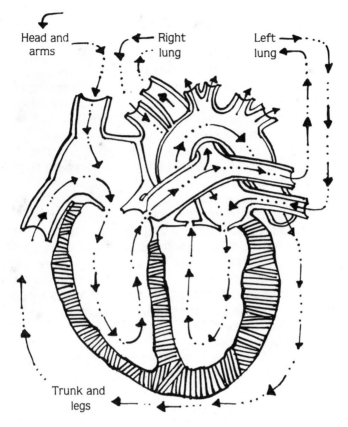

Figure 3   The blood circulation

of four pulmonary veins and emptied into the *left* atrium of the heart. It then proceeds into the left ventricle which, on contraction, pumps the blood into the *aorta* (main artery) which supplies organs and other structures by means of several branches.

In the region of the neck, one branch of the aorta — the *common carotid artery* — divides into internal and external arteries. The *external carotid* artery, you may recall, divides into three main branches to supply the outer part of the skull and the face (see Chapter 3, p. 27).

Arteries divide into many smaller branches (arterioles) which, in turn, subdivide into even smaller vessels (capillaries). Hair on the head is fed by the capillaries supplying the papillae in the subsurface layer of the scalp. It is through the medulla or inner layer that hair absorbs the nutrients brought to it by these minute blood vessels, as mentioned in Chapter 3, p. 29.

Some of those persons who specialize in hair transplants and other such invasive hair replacement procedures scoff at the fact that decreased blood supply is a contributing cause of abnormal hair loss. One of these — a doctor whose speciality is hair transplant surgery, and who obviously would like to add to his clientele — has conceded, however (albeit reluctantly), that 'nutritionist theories' have not been disproven, and could possibly be right. He goes on to state that many people just do not eat the right food!

Those who do not subscribe to the fact that depriving the scalp of oxygen, through the blood supply, and of essential nutrients leads to hair loss, cite in their defence experiments carried out by the Belgian researcher, Dr Raymond Maréchal.

Dr Maréchal tied off some of the main blood vessels to the scalp of some 300 balding clients. This, of course, reduced the scalp's blood supply. The doctor reported that over 50 per cent of his clients stopped losing their hair, and that 21 per cent of them noted a retardation of the loss.

There is another side to this seemingly impressive anecdote, however. Within a year, authorities agree, the body creates a 'collateral' blood supply to compensate for what was tampered with. And that is why surgeons are not going around tying off their balding patients' scalp blood vessels. They are aware that the apparent success of such a procedure would be, at best, temporary only.

The body is wiser than we give it credit for. It will struggle to survive and to function as intended — the reason why it develops compensatory mechanisms when the original is interfered with. It makes a supreme effort to carry out its natural functions, regardless of injury or invasion. That is why we develop fevers, inflammation and swelling — to combat invading organisms. That is why the scalp develops a collateral blood supply — because it is so vital!

The food we eat

The food we take into our bodies is composed of proteins, carbohydrates, fats, water, fibre and a host of vitamins and minerals. It is important from the outset to be aware that all these elements work together and that, as a general rule, no one, in isolation, will produce miraculous results.

Proteins

Proteins form the basic structure of every living body cell: your hair, skin, eyes and nails are essentially protein. (The three layers of which individual hairs are made up, you will recollect, are held together by a mesh that is largely protein.)

The best animal sources of protein are lean meat, poultry and fish, milk and its byproducts, and eggs.

Vegetable protein sources include grains (such as corn, oats and wheat) and legumes (dried peas, beans and lentils), but in order to be complete, they must be correctly combined at the same meal with a complementary protein.

For further information on protein complementarity, I suggest that you read *Diet for a Small Planet* by Frances Moore Lappé.

Carbohydrates

Carbohydrates (starches and sugars) are the most common source of our food energy. The best carbohydrate sources include whole grains, fresh fruits and fresh vegetables.

Fats

Fats (lipids) are necessary for energy, for conserving heat and for the proper functioning of all body cells. Unsaturated fats in the diet are considered very beneficial for the health of the sebaceous glands which produce lubrication for the scalp and hair and moisturizer for the skin.

The best food sources of fats are unrefined oils from vegetables, nuts and seeds (such as olives, peanuts, safflower, corn, sesame seeds, sunflower seeds and soy beans) and from raw seeds, nuts, milk and milk products.

Water

The human body is about 50 per cent water. Water is a major constituent of blood, lymph and cells, and it is the medium through which essential nutrients are transported wherever required. Most foods contain water.

Fibre

Fibre (indigestible carbohydrate, cellulose, roughage or bulk), formerly thought of as having no value in the diet, is now regarded by many doctors and researchers as very important indeed to wellbeing.

Studies persuasively indicate that there is a much lower incidence of disorders like varicose veins, blood clots, high cholesterol level, atherosclerosis and obesity among people whose diet is high in fibre than in those whose diet is deficient in this material. Certainly, fibre is important for proper elimination of waste matter from the body.

The best source of fibre is natural wheat bran (not to be confused with *All Bran*). It is inexpensive and can be added to breakfast cereals and juices, or incorporated into home cooking (such as baked foods and casseroles).

Other good sources of fibre are unrefined whole grains, berries (such as blackberries and raspberries), dates, black and lima beans, almonds (eaten fresh from the shell), potatoes in their jacket and corn.

Vitamins

In his book, *New Hope for Your Hair*, Dr Irwin I. Lubowe, a well-known American dermatologist, points out that the effects on the growth of hair caused by vitamin deficiency (and in at least one instance, vitamin excess) have been demonstrated so often by researchers that we must consider these findings with the utmost seriousness. He goes on to observe that many people simply are not eating as they should.

With these facts in mind, therefore, let us take a look at the role of vitamins, and later minerals (pp. 46-50), on the health and life of scalp hair.

Vitamins are, as the name suggests, life-giving substances that are needed, usually in small amounts, for health and growth.

Vitamin A

Vitamin A is a fat-soluble vitamin needed to build resistance to infection, for healthy skin, hair and mucous membrane (lining body cavities, like the mouth), and for healthy gums, teeth, eyes and glands.

Vitamin A is obtained, ready-made, from foods of animal origin, and from plant sources in the form of carotene, which is turned into the vitamin in the body.

Fresh vegetables highest in this nutrient are carrots,

dandelion leaves, endive, parsley, sweet potatoes and turnip greens. Fresh fruits yielding the most vitamin A are apricots, cantaloupe melons, cherries, mangoes, mulberries, nectarines, papayas and peaches.

Other vitamin A sources are fish liver oils, eggs, dairy products, fish and meats.

An *excessive* intake of vitamin A, however, is detrimental to the hair and skin; drying of the skin, inflammation of the hair follicles and baldness could result. These conditions, however, are reversible once the dosage of the vitamin taken is reduced to normal.

Vitamin C

Vitamin C (ascorbic acid) is a water-soluble vitamin needed for healthy tissues, for healing and to reinforce the body's resistance to disease. It is essential for the maintenance of collagen, the cement-like substance that holds cells together. It assists in blood circulation and oxygen utilization.

Since our bodies cannot make (synthesize) this vitamin, we must obtain it each day from food sources in order to preserve good health.

The best vegetable sources of vitamin C are cabbage, green and red peppers, dandelion leaves, kohlrabi, mustard and cress and turnip tops, although almost all fresh vegetables, particularly if eaten raw, will contribute to your vitamin C intake.

The best fresh fruit sources of this nutrient are apricots, blackberries, cantaloupe melons, cherries, elderberries, gooseberries, grapefruit, guavas, honeydew melon, kumquats, lemons, limes, oranges, papaya, redcurrants, rosehips and strawberries.

Vitamin D

Vitamin D is a fat-soluble vitamin needed for the proper assimilation of other nutrients from the digestive tract. The body uses this vitamin in the transportation of oxygen from one part to another. Some experts believe that not even a 'normal' diet provides sufficient vitamin D.

Some vitamin D may be obtained from liver, milk and egg yolk, also from fish and seafood and from several of the foods that furnish vitamin A. The best sources of this nutrient, however, are fish liver oils and sunlight (through its action on the skin).

Vitamin E
Vitamin E is a fat-soluble vitamin that is noted for its role in regulating the body's oxygen supplies and maintaining the efficiency of the blood circulation. A vitamin E deficiency may cause increased fragility of the red blood cells.

Good vitamin E sources include whole grains, legumes, seeds, nuts, green leafy vegetables, fruits, eggs, beef liver and unrefined vegetable oils.

Vitamin F
Vitamin F (essential fatty acids) come under the heading of 'fats'. One of these acids (linoleic acid) is vital to body functioning. Polyunsaturated fats such as unrefined oils can supply this nutrient; so can nuts (especially almonds and walnuts) and fish.

Vitamin K
Vitamin K (the 'blood vitamin') is a fat-soluble vitamin which, by helping the blood to clot readily, counteracts any tendency to excessive bleeding. It assists the liver in its vital functions and helps in the utilization of vitamin E.

Prime sources of vitamin K are green leafy vegetables, alfalfa sprouts, pork liver, unrefined vegetable oils, egg yolk, cow's milk, tomatoes, soy beans and wheatgerm.

5.

THE VITAL HAIR NUTRIENTS

Because they are indispensable to vigorous hair growth, the B vitamins, sometimes called the 'nerve vitamins', deserve a separate chapter to themselves.

✳ The B vitamins

The B vitamins are a complex of over a dozen water-soluble vitamins that are notable for helping in the maintenance of energy reserves and for fighting stress. They help in the building and repair of body cells, including the red blood cells. They include thiamin (B_1), riboflavin (B_2), niacin (B_3), pyridoxine (B_6), folic acid (B_9) and cyanocobalamin (B_{12}).

Thiamin

Thiamin (B_1) enables body cells to obtain energy from the nutrients brought to them by the blood. This vitamin cannot be stored, and so a daily supply is essential. Thiamin, moreover, is vital to important body functions like muscle contraction, blood circulation, digestion and nervous system activity.

Scientific studies indicate that a thiamin-deficient diet may adversely affect hair growth. When laboratory animals were deprived of this nutrient for a few weeks, they developed altered hair cycles and ragged-looking fur and showed evidence of hair loss. Resumption of a normal diet, however, corrected these unfavourable signs.

The richest sources of thiamin are lean pork, heart, liver, kidney, nutritional yeast, whole grains and raw nuts and seeds. Other sources include legumes, green leafy vegetables and potatoes.

Riboflavin

Riboflavin (B_2) is essential for health and growth. It helps in the transportation of oxygen from one part of the body to another. It aids the metabolism and assimilation of carbohydrate.

A shortage of riboflavin in the diet can lead to skin disorders, dryness and cracking of the corners of the mouth, impaired nerve function, increased vulnerability to infection and generalized fatigue and weakness.

Foods high in riboflavin include liver, kidney, heart, beef, chicken, milk and milk products, eggs, green leafy vegetables, broccoli, whole grains, legumes, lima beans, nutritional yeast and sunflower seeds.

Niacin

Niacin (B_3) helps to maintain good blood circulation and a healthy nervous system and skin. It also aids in the assimilation of carbohydrates. A niacin-deficient diet could lead to dermatitis (skin inflammation), loss of memory and swelling of certain tissues (such as the gums).

Good food sources of niacin are whole grains, seeds, legumes, nuts, green leafy vegetables, potatoes, asparagus, artichoke, fish, lamb, offal like liver and kidneys and nutritional yeast.

Pyridoxine

Pyridoxine (B_6) plays a major role in the body's utilization of proteins, carbohydrates and fats in the normal functioning of skin, muscles and nerves, as well as in the production of the hormones adrenaline and insulin. A pyridoxine deficiency may lead to nervousness, insomnia and nausea. Experimental animals fed a diet lacking this nutrient showed signs of hair loss and scaly, inflamed skin.

Good sources of pyridoxine include legumes, carrots, cabbage, avocados, bananas, prunes, raisins, beef, liver, kidney, pork, whole grains, eggs, fresh fish, milk, nuts (such as pecans and walnuts), sunflower seeds and nutritional yeast.

Folic acid

Folic acid (B_9) is vital to the formation of healthy red blood cells and for keeping the body's natural defence system working efficiently. It helps to maintain proper liver function and to utilize fats.

Deficiency of folic acid may cause various forms of anaemia. It can adversely affect healing ability and may cause hair (including eyebrows and eyelashes) to fall out. It may also be a factor influencing the maintenance and restoration of normal hair colour.

The richest food sources of folic acid are dark green leafy vegetables, nuts, liver and nutritional yeast.

Cyanocobalamin

Cyanocobalamin (B_{12}) possesses an anti-anaemic factor (preventing anaemia or 'iron-poor blood') and is essential for the formation and regeneration of normal blood cells and for satisfactory nerve function. Deficiency, of course, can lead to anaemia.

The best food sources of this nutrient are liver, milk, lean meats, eggs, nutritional yeast, cheese and wheatgerm.

Anti-stress vitamins

Associated with the B-complex group of vitamins are other nutrients which have been linked with the health of the hair (three of these are known as the *anti-stress vitamins*).

Biotin

Biotin stimulates cell growth. In experimental animals, deficiency of this nutrient caused inflammation of the skin and greying and falling of the hair to the point of baldness. Dr Irwin I. Lubowe has remarked that this may be an important supplement.

The late Adelle Davis, one of America's best known nutritionists, has cautioned against the regular use of raw egg white. Avidin, she pointed out, a substance in raw egg white, can combine with biotin in the intestine and prevent it from reaching the blood.

Half a cup of powdered, uncooked egg white was added to an adequate diet and fed to human volunteers. The subjects developed dry, peeling skin and other untoward signs and symptoms. When biotin was added to the diet, however, all the symptoms disappeared within five days.

The prime food sources of biotin are nutritional yeast, liver, eggs, whole grains, fish, desiccated liver and wheatgerm.

Para-aminobenzoic acid

Para-aminobenzoic acid (PABA) was first publicized as an anti-grey hair vitamin because black animals deficient in the nutrient developed grey hair. When these animals were fed the vitamin, normal hair colour was restored.

Furthermore, Dr Benjamin Sieve, a Boston nutritionist, made exhaustive studies of the hair of persons given 200mg of PABA after each meal. In 70 per cent of the cases, some hair regained its natural colour.

Deficiency of PABA, biotin, folic acid and pantothenic acid (see below) appears to affect hair colour. One scientist who did research on the B vitamins for many years has repeatedly produced grey hair in dark-haired animals.

Adelle Davis has remarked that normal hair colour is rarely restored by taking synthetic B vitamins. But she has witnessed temporary restoration of normal hair colour in persons who regularly took a diet rich in the B vitamins. Even when no effect on hair colour was demonstrated, the hair improved in quality and vigour of growth when these nutrients were faithfully included in the diet.

PABA, like the other vitamins in this complex, is supplied by foods such as liver, kidney, eggs, whole grains, molasses and nutritional yeast, liver being the richest source.

Inositol

Inositol is a compound occurring in the brain, muscles, liver, kidneys and lens of the eye.

In laboratory animals, a diet lacking inositol produced baldness. But when the vitamin was added to the food, the hair grew again. Moreover, it was observed that male animals lost hair twice as fast as females. This suggested that males require a higher inositol intake than females. An inositol deficiency also causes eczema, a form of skin irritation.

It is interesting to note that, with the exception of niacin, inositol occurs in the human body almost a hundred times more than any other vitamin.

Noteworthy, too, is that of all the B vitamins, only inositol markedly increased the contractions of the eliminatory tract of the body (such as the intestines) when these nutrients were given in barium (a radio-opaque substance) to volunteers, and the results studied through a fluoroscope. This may well be significant in the treatment of constipation, a condition best avoided if superb health is desired. And we must never lose sight of the fact that the health of the hair and scalp are inextricably bound up with the health of the rest of the body.

Many years ago when Adelle Davis became interested in the possible connection between inositol in the diet (or lack of it) and hair loss, she recommended it, together with other sources of the B vitamins, to all the bald men who consulted her. In almost every case, hair loss was arrested. In some cases, new hair growth was evident in as little as one month. In one striking case, a man who had been bald since the age of twenty completely recovered his lost hair so that not one bald spot remained!

Inositol, too, appears to reduce the amount of cholesterol in the blood.

Inositol and the cholesterol connection

Cholesterol is a fat-like material found in many places of the body (such as nerve tissue of the brain and spinal cord and in the blood). Our bodies need it (for example, to produce bile and for metabolism), but too much is undesirable. The surplus tends to stick to the inner walls of blood vessels (for instance, arteries), and this could result in *atherosclerosis,* a condition in which blobs of fatty and other material build up within the arteries, making them thick and hard, reducing their elasticity and *narrowing the channel for the efficient flow of blood.*

Cholesterol deposits may, therefore, affect the blood vessels of the scalp, just as they do other blood vessels of the body. As these vessels become narrower, the blood circulation is proportionately restricted so that nutrients essential to the health and life of the hair cells do not reach the hair bulbs and the papillae, which are the hair's manufacturing plant.

Researchers have tried to attack cholesterol build-up so as to give added diameter to the blood vessels and improve the blood flow. They have used various vasodilators, agents which literally dilate or widen the vessels, in an effort to produce the desired effect. But, as with the prolonged use of any medication, long-term use of vasodilators does produce undesirable side-effects, and the most sensible long-range approach to keeping blood vessels patent appears to be a reduction of cholesterol deposits through proper diet. This can be successfully achieved, to a large extent, by reducing the consumption of highly saturated fats (of animal origin), salt and refined sugar, and by increasing fibre intake.

The best inositol sources are liver and nutritional yeast; but fresh fruits and vegetables, whole grains, nuts and seeds, legumes, lean meats, milk and dark, unrefined molasses are commendable sources.

Choline and lecithin

Choline acts with inositol and forms part of the structure of lecithin, a substance produced by the liver and found in the brain in large amounts. It is part of the protective covering of nerves (the myelin sheath).

Lecithin helps to keep cholesterol particles tiny so that they can be readily utilized by the tissues. It helps in the digestion and absorption of fats and of vitamins A, D, E and K (the fat-soluble vitamins).

When young experimental animals were fed a choline-deficient diet, their blood pressure became high and their blood cholesterol level skyrocketed. Choline deficiency, by restricting the synthesis of lecithin, causes cholesterol to build up and clog blood vessels. Stepping up the choline content of the diet can contribute to a lowering of the blood cholesterol level.

In a study made of 158 persons with very high blood pressure, choline administration effected a normal, or near-normal, level in almost all cases: blood vessels dilated — as they did in experimental animals — to permit better blood flow under less pressure.

The richest sources of choline are liver, brains, nutritional yeast, egg yolk, kidneys, fish, peanuts and soy beans.

Pantothenic acid

Pantothenic acid (B_5), also known as calcium pantothenate, is considered an anti-dermatitis factor, important to the health of the skin. Pantothenic acid is necessary for the wellbeing of every body cell, and neither carbohydrate nor fat can be changed into energy without it.

This nutrient is also important for the normal functioning of the adrenal glands (located just above the kidneys) which produce much of the male's sex hormones, and for proper digestion. In human volunteers in whom pantothenic acid deficiencies were produced, increased vulnerability to infection was noted, as was adrenal exhaustion. Blood pressure dropped below normal and constipation developed.

In animals which lack this nutrient, the hair becomes grey and the hair bulbs and follicles atrophy (waste away). Pantothenic acid deficiency also appears to contribute to allergies and to low blood sugar.

This nutrient may be obtained from liver, heart, kidney, lean beef, egg yolk, whole grains, green vegetables, nutritional yeast, molasses, peanuts, sunflower seeds, broccoli, cabbage, corn, milk, potatoes, salmon, and unrefined vegetable oils.

6.

ESSENTIAL HAIR MINERALS

Minerals are essential constituents of all body cells. They are necessary for the normal functioning of all systems.

The body's mineral needs

Calcium
Calcium is needed for the proper functioning of nervous tissue, and for the normal clotting of blood. It is considered an anti-stress mineral, and it is needed to help maintain a sound chemical balance in the body.

High-calcium foods include vegetables (broccoli, Chinese cabbage, dandelion leaves, kale, mustard and cress, parsley, spinach, turnip greens and watercress), legumes, citrus fruits, dried figs, milk and milk products, carob flour and molasses.

Iron
Iron is a vital component of haemoglobin (the red colouring matter of blood), which transports oxygen to every cell in the body. An iron deficiency results in anaemia.

The richest natural sources of iron are vegetables (chard (spinach), dandelion and mustard and cress, green leafy vegetables and parsley), legumes, seaweed, dried fruits (notably prunes and raisins), persimmons, watermelon, lean beef, heart, kidney, liver (especially pork liver), liver sausage, whole grains (buckwheat, millet, oats, rice), sesame seeds, molasses, egg yolk, nutritional yeast and sardines.

Magnesium

Magnesium, along with phosphorus, helps other body cells to utilize nutrients properly. It is necessary for good nervous control of muscles, and is important in calcium and phosphorus metabolism.

Good sources of this nutrient are whole grains, milk, citrus fruits, dried fruits, nuts, seeds, dark green leafy vegetables, liver, legumes, egg yolk, potatoes, tomatoes and coconut.

Phosphorus

Phosphorus is vital to the life processes of every body cell. It is abundant in the adrenal gland cells.

Adelle Davis has remarked that phosphorus is possibly more important than any other mineral in the body, but that it is usually overabundant in the diet.

Notable phosphorus sources are milk and milk products, eggs, poultry, lean meats, fish, nuts, seeds, whole grains and all unrefined foods.

Iodine

Iodine is needed by the thyroid gland to manufacture thyroxine, a hormone influencing many body functions. It is found in high concentration in the cortex (outer portion) of the adrenal glands. Lack of iodine can cause anaemia and premature greying and poor quality hair, or abnormal hair loss.

Good food sources of iodine are seaweed, seafood, sea fish, onions, garlic, cabbage, carrots, broccoli, lettuce, pineapple, foods grown in iodine-rich seacoast soils, eggs, oatmeal and unpeeled potatoes (new or potatoes baked in their jackets).

Potassium

Potassium is important for the maintenance of the body's acid-base balance and for the equilibrium of body fluids. It is needed for good nerves, and works with calcium to help counteract stress.

Potassium also contributes to the efficiency of the body's waste disposal system through its effect on the glands. High blood pressure has been produced in human volunteers by a potassium-deficient diet.

Potassium is usually richly supplied in the diet; but the common practice of soaking and boiling vegetables and discarding the water contributes to a pitiful waste of this important nutrient.

The best sources of potassium are fruits and vegetables, molasses, legumes, lean meats, fish, seaweed, nuts, unrefined grains, seeds, nutritional yeast, all citrus fruits, watercress, mint leaves, green peppers, alfalfa tea and sea plants (such as kelp).

Silicon

Silicon, according to some experts, gives beautiful finishing touches to the body, life to the skin and beauty to the hair. Silicon is required for healthy connective tissue and for the normal functioning of the adrenal glands.

All foods made from natural buckwheat are particularly rich in this nutrient, but other good sources are asparagus, carrots, celery, green pepper, lettuce, parsley, pumpkin, tomatoes, eggs, strawberries, oats and other whole grains, mushrooms, liver and lentils.

Sodium

Sodium (salt) is required for a normal fluid balance in the tissues. It is needed by the adrenal glands to function properly and for good digestion. It helps to purify the blood and is an essential part of muscle tissue.

Sodium works with two other elements (potassium and chlorine) to attract nutrients from the intestines into the blood, and from the blood into the cells, by maintaining what is known as 'osmotic pressure'.

Sodium is abundant in the diet, but the best sources are those occurring naturally in unrefined foods. These include asparagus, beet greens, beets, cabbage, carrots, celery, lima beans, pumpkin, spinach, prunes, strawberries, milk and milk products, fish, lean meats, poultry and whole wheat.

Trace minerals

Apart from the foregoing minerals, there is a group known as 'trace minerals', which are needed in the diet in very small amounts only.

Cobalt

Cobalt helps to prevent a certain type of anaemia (pernicious anaemia). Some years ago, thousands of animals grazing on land deficient in cobalt (for example, in Florida and Australia) became very ill and died from anaemia.

Cobalt is supplied by seafoods, seaweed (such as kelp), liver, green leafy vegetables, egg yolk, mushrooms, lentils, buckwheat and carrots.

Copper

Copper plays a role in the makeup of every body cell. It helps in the development and function of brain, nerves and connective tissue. A copper deficiency in the diet prevents the red blood cells from absorbing iron and so shortens their lifespan, resulting in anaemia.

In animals, a lack of copper manifests itself in skin rash, hair loss and degeneration of the myelin sheath which covers the nerves.

Copper also plays a part in the formation of hair colouring: black animals deficient in this nutrient become grey. In humans, too, anaemia (and copper deficiency contributing to it) has long been associated with greying.

The richest sources of copper are liver, kidney and brain. Other sources include legumes, molasses, whole grains, green leafy vegetables, black figs, oysters, almonds, apricots, figs, loganberries, walnuts, molasses and egg yolk.

Zinc

Zinc plays an important role in many body functions and zinc deficiency in humans is more widespread than recognized.

In severely burned persons, dietary zinc supplements produced rapid healing. Blood cholesterol levels dropped in patients with a high cholesterol build-up in their arteries.

In countries where severe zinc deficiencies occur (such as Egypt and Iran), sexual development is adversely affected.

Rich sources of zinc are fish, shellfish (especially oysters), nuts, whole grains, seeds, green leafy vegetables, fruits, eggs, liver, nutritional yeast, lean beef, pork, lamb and raw carrots.

Manganese

Manganese is known as a tissue strengthener. Good food sources include egg yolk, parsley, watercress, chives, almonds, walnuts, whole wheat and green leafy vegetables.

Selenium

Selenium is needed for the maintenance of the blood

circulatory system, to reinforce the body's natural defence mechanism and for virility. It works with vitamins C and E to help detoxify the body. Its deficiency has been linked with high blood pressure and premature ageing.

Good selenium sources are nutritional yeast, garlic, whole grains, asparagus, mushrooms, eggs and seafood.

Why we need nutrients

It is important to recognize the close relationship existing between the health of the scalp and hair and that of the rest of the body. When the general condition of the body is poor or fair only, its resistance to infection is lowered and its functioning is suboptimal. And so it is with the scalp and hair, which are part of the whole body.

All body cells depend on a healthful and rich supply of health-giving and life-giving nutrients for their wellbeing and vitality. These nutrients are brought to them by the bloodstream, and if the quality of this blood supply is poor, if the vessels making up the blood circulatory system are clogged or otherwise defective, then the tissues they feed will manifest this poverty. This, of course, includes the scalp in which the hair is housed. Poorly fed, the scalp will languish. The hair will lack lustre, be brittle and eventually part company with its 'roots', perhaps permanently.

The foregoing observations are very much in accord with what responsible researchers have noted. One of them, Dr Roger Williams, points out that cells in hair follicles will produce hair when they are *furnished with everything they need* (my emphasis). But, he asserts, in the scalp of a balding person, they *do not* get everything they need! He believes that this is probably because of faulty blood circulation so that, as a result, the hair-producing cells gradually die. Dr Williams considers this a sort of 'disease' process caused by cellular malnutrition.

We are fortunate to have such a rich variety of health-promoting foods at our disposal. We have only to be knowledgeable as to what substances they contain, why these substances are essential for the optimal health of hair and scalp and body, and how best to incorporate them into our diets.

Heredity

People are quick to use 'heredity' as the scapegoat for progressive hair loss. And yet, although the heredity factor does undoubtedly play a part, one has only to compare photos in family albums of yesteryear with those of today: our forebears, for the most part, displayed more hirsute heads than many of us now do. We seem to be losing our hair faster, and at a younger age, than they did. And as I mentioned in the Introduction of this book, experts predict the possibility of a generation of bald-pated men in the next century because of certain trends.

A possible and persuasive explanation is that our ancestors ate foods in a far more natural a state than we do, and that these foods were grown on nutrient-rich soils, unlike those cultivated in many places today. They very likely obtained a diet richer in natural minerals, vitamins and other hair-sustaining nutrients than we now do.

Let us not, therefore, for our hair's sake, waste more nutrients than we have to. The food processors and manufacturers do enough of that already. To help you, therefore, to conserve and utilize all the vitamins, minerals and other essential elements in the food you purchase to fuel your body and the hair it produces, and keep them healthy and vital, here are some invaluable suggestions.

Buying, storing and preparing food

The food you purchase will do you (and your hair) no good if it is improperly handled, stored and cooked or otherwise prepared.

Storage
Vegetables are best stored at cool temperatures (such as in a pantry or refrigerator) to prevent the action of enzymes that destroy nutrients.

Green leafy vegetables lose much of their thiamin (B_1) and vitamin C if left at room temperature for even one day.

Fruits with thick skins (such as oranges, bananas, melons and pineapples) may be kept at room temperatures. But ripe fruits should be refrigerated promptly if they are to retain their vitamins A, B-complex and C. Guavas, for instance, which are exceedingly rich in vitamin C (they contain up to 2000mg of vitamin C for every 454g, 1 lb) lose as much as four-fifths of this nutrient after standing at room temperature for one day.

Meats for long-term use are best stored in the freezer. Express as much air from the package to prevent deterioration. Meats to be used in a day may be kept in the coldest part of the refrigerator. Exposed to light (for example when thawing), meats lose much of their riboflavin (B_2).

The above tips for meat storage generally apply also to poultry and fish.

Legumes keep for about a year at room temperature. Store them in containers with tightfitting lids, away from sources of heat and moisture. Grains, too, are usually stored in this way.

Milk and milk products are, of course, best refrigerated. The riboflavin (B_2) they contain would soon be lost were they to be exposed to light (for example, milk is sold in glass bottles in some health food stores and kept in coolers with transparent doors).

Cheese for long-range use may be securely wrapped and frozen. Freezing, however, does render it crumbly, although this matters little if the product is to be used in salads or in cooking.

Eggs should be refrigerated promptly after purchase. They are best kept in the container in which they are bought as they are porous and easily admit the flavours of other foods, as well as bacteria. For these reasons, never wash eggs before storing them. Make sure that the larger side of the egg is uppermost. This keeps the yolk centred and the egg less vulnerable to contamination.

Bread for long-term use may be securely wrapped and stored in the freezer. For immediate use, bread is best kept in plastic bags in a bread box. In hot, humid weather it may be refrigerated.

Whole grain flours are best refrigerated or kept in some other cool place because they contain the germ of the grains — the most perishable part. Stored in warmer temperatures, these flours may become rancid. Rancidity hastens destruction of vitamins A, C, E and several B vitamins.

For the above reasons, also refrigerate oils (except olive and peanut, which become cloudy when stored at cooler temperatures).

Cooking utensils

You may, or may not, habitually prepare your own meals. If your wife or husband or other friend usually does this for you, please ask her or him to study this chapter carefully and to try to follow its suggestions faithfully. By doing so, the person in charge of most of your meal preparation will be contributing, in no small way, to the life and health of your hair.

Glassware is a slow conductor of heat and contributes to the destruction of riboflavin by admitting light.

Aluminium is a matter of choice. Some experts say that it is best avoided because small quantities of the aluminium oxide, which is potentially harmful to humans, dissolve into the food. Others reassure us that aluminium is insoluble and that we can safely cook in utensils made of it.

Cooking in cast-iron equipment can contribute a little iron to your dietary intake of this mineral. However, do not cook in pots and pans lined with copper, as food coming into direct contact with this metal quickly loses its nutrients through oxidation.

Food preparation

The sooner you are aware that exposure to air and light, and the subjection to high temperatures rob food of health-promoting properties, the sooner you will exercise care in preparing and cooking it.

When you learn that valuable nutrients lie directly under the skin of fruits and vegetables, you will eat these *with* the skins whenever practicable, and you will discard the potato peeler and use the paring knife more discriminately.

When you understand that soaking and draining vegetables leach precious minerals and vitamins and other nutrients from them, you will ignore recipe instructions that encourage you to waste so willfully.

Scrub potatoes and carrots and similar vegetables with a suitable scrubbing brush, under cold running water. Cook them with the skins intact; eat the skins whenever manageable. Wash salad greens, too, under cold running water. Do so quickly but thoroughly and shake them dry before use or storage. I put my salad greens in a pillowcase reserved for this purpose. I go onto my porch and swirl the case to expel the water clinging to the greens. I then put everything in the refrigerator until I am ready to prepare the salad. If the greens are more than I need at the moment, I put the surplus in a plastic container so that when it is time to make another salad, the greens are already clean and crisp.

Vegetables should be cut so as to expose to the air as little surface area as possible. For example, carrots cut lengthwise lose fewer nutrients than those chopped into small pieces.

When the vegetables are ready to be cooked, put them in a preheated pot of suitable size, with a minimum of liquid. Cover the utensil and reduce the heat at the first sign of vapour. The high initial heat inhibits the action of the vitamin C-destructive enzyme; the subsequent low heat helps to conserve health-promoting substances while rendering the food digestible and palatable.

Try not to lift the lid during cooking; it introduces air which destroys nutrients. Let the food cook only long enough to produce a tender vegetable.

Use any liquid left in the pot in a sauce, gravy, soup, stew or pancake or waffle batter, as it is rich in minerals and vitamins.

Best cooking methods

The cooking methods that best preserve the hair-regenerating properties in the food you buy are baking, grilling, pressure cooking, roasting, steaming and stir-frying. Any good cooking manual will describe how these are done. An authoritative Oriental cookbook will instruct you in the stir-fry technique.

Miscellaneous beverages

In developed and developing nations, tea and coffee are not to be denied most people. Nor are colas or chocolate and cocoa drinks. It is as well to know, however, that these beverages contain caffeine which is a diuretic, that is, an agent that promotes the excretion of water from the body.

Diuretics have been of some value in controlling hair loss to the extent that they help to excrete salt from the tissues.

(Too much salt in the diet is bad for the hair because it causes the body to retain water, especially in the scalp tissues. A high salt intake will contribute to conditions that are known to encourage hair loss, such as dandruff. It will help to create a better medium for scalp bacteria to thrive in. An excess of salt, in short, will aggravate hair loss.)

Dr Eugene Foldes of New York has carried out experiments

to show that people with a high salt content in their tissues demonstrated evidence of abnormal hair loss. When they used diuretics, however, there was noticeable improvement in the condition. Diuretics, though, also cause the elimination from the body of important nutrients such as potassium along with the water.

The wiser approach to keeping the salt intake low is to eat a wholesome diet that is low in sodium (salt) in the first place (see sections on sodium, pp. 48, 57-59).

The best beverages for habitual consumption are milk, unsweetened fruit juices, vegetable juices without added salt, herbal teas and, of course, water.

Alcohol

Alcohol has become an integral part of social life for many of us. In small amounts, alcohol is not bad.

Alcohol is a *vasodilator*, that is, it helps to give added diameter to blood vessels, relieving constriction and so improving blood flow to tissues throughout the body. But too much of a good thing is bad, just as two negatives do not make a positive, and alcohol abuse will be deleterious to the whole system — which includes the scalp and the hair.

It would be far better to keep blood vessels patent by dietary measures (for example, discouraging cholesterol buildup), such as suggested earlier in Chapter 5 (p. 43), and by the daily practice of relaxation techniques (see Chapter 10) which help to counteract the tension that constricts blood vessels.

Recipe: Banana shake

Into an electric blender, put 250ml (1 cup) whole liquid milk, 15-30ml (1-2 tablespoons) powdered milk and one ripe peeled banana broken into large pieces.

Cover the blender and liquefy the ingredients (about 10 seconds). Uncover the blender; add 5ml (1 teaspoon) unpasteurized honey. Again cover the blender and blend the contents for a further ten seconds. Pour the 'shake' into a large glass.

This recipe provides protein, minerals and vitamins. Because it is quick to make, it is an excellent quick breakfast drink for very busy persons, and a fast 'pick-me-up' for those times when the blood sugar level is low and energy flags.

Variation

Vary this recipe by omitting the banana and substituting any ripe fruit in season (remove large seeds), such as apricot, peach, strawberries or raspberries. The nutrient value of the 'shake' will then be determined by the nutrients contained in the specific fruit(s).

7.
A DIET PLAN FOR
HEALTHY HAIR REGENERATION

Some years ago, Dr Eugene Foldes (see p. 55) impressively demonstrated that a reduction of the salt content of the diet not only slowed down hair loss but even helped to reverse it. Unlike many other approaches to this problem, the 'desalting' of the body's tissues effected continued cessation of hair loss and in some cases positive recovery.

But Dr Foldes's experiments relied on the use of diuretics, agents that increase the excretion of water (through urination) from the body. And diuretics, like most medications used over a long period, tend to produce unsalutary side-effects.

Concerned experts agree, therefore, that the best way to keep the salt content of body tissues low is to adhere to a low-salt diet.

Why a low-salt diet?

High-salt diets have been linked to hypertension (high blood pressure) and, indeed, in countries where the diet is very high in salt (such as Japan), hypertension is commonplace.

Hypertension promotes heart disease. Because the blood has to course through blood vessels at greater than normal pressure, it places strain on the heart. Structures at the extremities of the body (such as the scalp) are consequently shortchanged of an adequate blood supply because the blood has to labour to reach its destination.

In a nutshell, a high-salt diet is an impediment to a healthy blood circulation, which is the life force behind healthy hair growth and hair renewal.

Many of us consume twenty to fifty times the amount of salt (sodium) actually needed daily. We tend to use the salt shaker far too liberally for our own good.

Most foods contain their own natural salt. The habit of adding salt to the cooking, or at the table to cooked food, should be quickly dropped. It is surely better to shed the salt-adding habit than shed the hair.

How to reduce your salt intake

1. Substitute herbs in your cooking for the usual salt. You'll find culinary herbs at your supermarket and in specialty stores. Examples of such herbs are: basil, bouquet garni, celery seed, chervil, chives, coriander, cumin, dill, fennel, fines herbes, marjoram, mint, oregano, paprika, parsley, rosemary, saffron, savory, tarragon and thyme.

   Herb charts are available in some stores. These tell you which herbs have an affinity for which dishes and best enhance them. Some cookbooks, too, introduce you to the delights of the world of herbs.

   You can grow some of these herbs easily in your own backyard, in a windowbox or in pots kept in or near the house. Ask at your local plant shop or herbalist, or check in your local library for a book on the subject.

2. Avoid using 'herb salts' (such as garlic salt and celery salt). They are too high in sodium. It is better to stick to the dried or fresh herbs.

3. Do not add salt to your food at the table; do not even put the salt shaker on the table.

4. Drastically reduce your consumption of cured meats (such as salami) and salted and smoked fish.

5. Severely restrict your intake of salty snacks such as potato chips, salted nuts and crackers and pickles.

6. Increase your intake of fresh fruits and vegetables (raw), nuts fresh from the shell, raw seeds (such as sesame and sunflower — you may lightly toast, but *not* salt, them), and whole grain, unsalted crackers and crispbreads.

7. Be a scrupulous label-reader when you go shopping. Some foods contain sodium, although they do not actually *taste* salty. Look for the words 'salt', 'sodium', and 'soda' on labels and avoid buying these products.

   Some compounds containing sodium include *monosodium glutamate* (MSG), a flavour-enhancer known to excite the nervous system unfavourably, and sodium bicarbonate (baking soda). Some types of baking powder

also contain sodium. Watch out for these.
8. Products marked 'made without salt', or 'no salt added'
    are not necessarily low in sodium. Again, read the
    ingredient listing on every product you pick up to decide
    whether you want to use it or not.

Why a low-fat diet?

We do need some fats (lipids) in the diet. Fats are required
for energy, to help conserve heat and for the proper
functioning of brain and other body cells (for example, the
hair cells). They are also needed for the production of the sex
and other hormones, and they are important for the
flourishing of valuable intestinal bacteria.

But we do not need *all* the fat we tend to consume — and
we do seem to consume a lot, as evidenced by the amount
of obesity and related conditions that are now widespread.

Best types of fat

Of the three types of fat (saturated, polyunsaturated and
monounsaturated), the second is, without question, the best
for health in general and for hair growth in particular.

Saturated fats
Saturated fats (which literally mean 'holding all that can be
absorbed, received or combined') tend to raise the cholesterol
concentration in the blood. Some even contain cholesterol.
These fats are of animal origin (for instance, whole dairy
products, lard, meat), and so constituted chemically as to be
incapable of absorbing additional hydrogen.

Polyunsaturated fats
Polyunsaturated fats, on the other hand, are those that help
the body to eliminate newly formed cholesterol. They
therefore help to reduce cholesterol build-up in the walls of
the arteries and to keep the level of cholesterol in the
bloodstream within normal limits.

Monounsaturated fats
Monounsaturated fats, though containing no cholesterol, do
not have the cholesterol-reducing properties of the
polyunsaturated fats.

To help to keep the blood fat level within normal limits, the American Heart Association recommends the incorporation of two to four tablespoons of liquid vegetable oil to the daily diet (for example, in a salad).

The most polyunsaturated oil is safflower. Soy bean, sunflower, corn and sesame oils follow in descending order. These vegetable oils are among the principal sources of essential fatty acids, substances imperative for healthy hair growth and restoration.

Storing oils
To prevent rancidity, which hastens the destruction of vitamin E, do refrigerate all your polyunsaturated oils.

More on cholesterol
In Chapter 5, I outlined what cholesterol is, where it is found and what it does. But it stands repeating that a high blood cholesterol level is a threat to an adequate blood supply to the scalp and hair. And according to the respected American dermatologist, Dr Irwin Lubowe, it cannot be emphasized often enough that *an adequate blood supply to scalp and hair is critical at a time of scalp disorder*, and, of course, important to general health and wellbeing.

Can cholesterol be controlled?
Experts say 'yes'. Foods that help to lower the blood cholesterol level include liquid vegetable oils (already mentioned), lean fish, poultry and low-fat milk.

Low-fat hints
1. Buy lean cuts of meat (such as fillet steak), lean fish (such as cod), chicken, turkey and rabbit more often than, say, lamb, pork and ham, which contain more fat than lean meat, gram for gram.
2. Be sparing in your use of cured meats (such as bacon, or liverwurst).
3. Buy only lean minced beef (83 per cent lean).
4. Read carefully labels on canned, packaged and bottled foods. Do not be misled by phrases like 'vegetable oil' or 'vegetable fat', which often mean 'saturated vegetable fat' (for instance, coconut or palm oil).
5. Trim fat from meats *before* cooking them.

6. Cool and refrigerate gravies, sauces, soups and stews; skim off the congealed surface fat; reheat and serve.
7. Bake, grill, steam or stir-fry foods rather than, say, fry or deep-fry them.

Why a low-sugar diet?

Because sugar (and I refer to refined sugar whenever I use this word) provides only empty calories. We can get the same energy, as well as useful nutrients, from a variety of natural, wholesome foods.

What is more, some persons are predisposed to form a high blood cholesterol level when their sugar consumption is high. Many people ingest over 45kg (100 lbs) of refined sugar a year through the consumption of prepared foods, pastries and other baked goods, and beverages.

Sweet nothings
Sweeteners of all kinds contribute to a malnutrition of the body's tissues by usurping the place in the diet rightfully belonging to more healthful foods. One tablespoon of sugar, for example, provides 25 calories.

Nutritionists advise not to programme the palate to expect and demand large quantities of sweeteners, low-calorie or non-calorie or otherwise.

Sugar is the arch-enemy of the B vitamins which, as we know, are probably the most vital of the vitamins to the survival and health of the hair. Sugar has little or no place in the diet of anyone wishing to keep the hair and keep it healthy.

Low-sugar tips
1. Be an avid label-reader. Be on the alert for imitation maple syrups, which are often cane or corn syrup with simulated maple flavouring added. Look also for 'hidden' sugars (for instance, sucrose, dextrose, lactose). Some cold breakfast cereals contain as much as 70 per cent sugar!
2. Ingredients of products are listed in descending order of quantity. For instance, if you buy a can of beans that reads: sugar, water, beans, salt, spices, sugar and water are major ingredients.
3. Wherever possible, substitute naturally dried fruits, fresh fruits, yogurt and raw nuts and seeds for cakes and

pastries, chocolate bars, rich toppings and candy.
4. Go easy on all sweeteners, honey included.

Why a high-fibre diet?

In Chapter 4, I explained what fibre is, why we need it, what are its best sources and how it can be incorporated into the diet.

In Chapter 11, I give additional and, I believe, convincing material regarding the importance of fibre in the diet. I observe, too, that most people in the so-called 'civilized' countries partake of a diet that is far too low in this ingredient.

Suffice it to mention here, then, only that in the interest of halting hair loss and possibly reversing it, you would do well to boost your dietary fibre intake.

The hair-diet plan in a nutshell

- Reduce your salt intake.
- Cut down your consumption of saturated fats.
- Restrict your ingestion of refined sugar.
- Increase your intake of fibre.
- Eat from a wide variety of wholesome, natural foods.
- Become a seasoned label-reader.

8.

HORMONES AND YOUR HAIR

Our endocrine glandular system influences everything we do and affects our very existence. Some even say that we are the product of our endocrine glands.

With this in mind, let us take a look at these glands, what they do and how they influence the health of our hair through their effect on the entire human organism.

Endocrine glands

Endocrine glands (from the Greek *endon*, within, and *krinein*, to secrete) are ductless glands of internal secretion that produce hormones (from the Greek *hormon*, urging on). These hormones are secreted directly into the blood or lymph for circulation to all parts of the body. They produce effects on tissues — even those remote from where the glands secreting them are located.

In addition to their endocrine function, some glands (such as the pancreas and the testes) also produce an external secretion.

The hormones secreted by the endocrine, or ductless, glands may have a specific effect on an organ or tissue, or a general effect on the entire body (for example, the thyroid gland affects the rate of metabolism).

Some endocrine glands produce a single hormone; others, such as the pituitary, produce several hormones.

Among the physiological processes affected by hormones are metabolic rate, metabolism of specific substances, growth and developmental processes, the secretory activity of other endocrine glands, nervous functions and the ability of the body to cope with conditions of stress and to resist disease.

Endocrine dysfunction may result from an undersecretion (hyposecretion) in which an insufficient amount of hormone(s) is produced, or an oversecretion (hypersecretion) in which excessive secretion takes place.

The secretion of the endocrine glands may be under the influence of chemical substances in the blood or, in some cases, under the control of other hormones (for example, those produced by the anterior lobe of the pituitary gland influence all the other endocrine glands).

Many pathological and other undesirable conditions are the result of, or associated with, the malfunctioning of the endocrine glands, and it is important from the outset to realize that all the glands in this system (as well as all the other systems of the body) work together for good or ill.

The pituitary gland (hypophysis)

Because it influences the activity of many other endocrine glands, the pituitary is called 'the master gland' or the 'conductor of the endocrine orchestra'.

It lies at the base of the skull, and consists of two lobes: an anterior (front) and posterior (back), as well as an intermediate part (pars intermedia).

The *anterior lobe* produces a number of *hormones which control the hormone production of all the other endocrine glands.* The significance of this fact will become more meaningful when you come to Chapter 9 and learn why exercises that invert the body are so important to vibrant hair growth.

Hormones produced by the pituitary

Among the hormones produced by the anterior pituitary are:

The *thyrotropic hormone,* which controls the activity of the thyroid gland in the production of thyroxin (see thyroid gland).

The *adrenotropic hormones,* which control the activity of the adrenal glands in the production of *cortin* (cortisone) from the cortex (outer portion) of the gland, and *adrenaline* from the medulla (central portion).

The *gonadotropic hormone,* which controls the activity of the male and female sex glands. In the female, it controls the internal secretions of the ovary (including the oestrogens and progesterone), and in the male it controls the activity of the testes in the production of male sex hormones.

The *posterior lobe* of the pituitary gland makes *pituitrin* which contains three factors. One of these, *vasopressin*, has an important influence on plain muscle fibre (for example, of the blood vessels). Another is an antidiuretic factor which influences the absorption of water by the kidneys.

The thyroid gland
The thyroid gland consists of two lobes lying one on each side of the windpipe (trachea). They are connected by a strip of thyroid substance (the isthmus).

The secretion of this gland *(thyroxine)* is regulated by the thyrotropic hormone secreted by the anterior pituitary and by the sympathetic nervous system.

According to Dr Steven Brena, author of *Yoga and Medicine*, modern endocrinology (study of the endocrine glands) teaches that the thyroid gland is a star of the first magnitude in the endocrine constellation and that improved function of the gland is translated into a general wellbeing of the entire human organism.

Thyroxine controls the body's entire metabolism and needs for its satisfactory manufacture a sufficient supply of iodine. Thyroxine also indirectly influences nutrition.

The parathyroid glands
These are four small glands placed two on each side of the thyroid gland.

Their secretion *(parathormone)* regulates calcium and phosphorus metabolism and controls the amount of calcium in the blood. Indirectly, parathormone affects muscular irritability.

The adrenal glands
These lie, one each, on the upper part of each kidney. They consist of an outer yellowish part (the cortex), which produces *cortin*, or *cortisone*, and an inner portion (the medulla) which produces *adrenaline*.

Cortisone influences carbohydrate metabolism, salt and water balance and muscle tone. It also exerts some effect on sexual characteristics.

Adrenaline
Adrenaline is constantly passing into the blood that richly

circulates in the adrenal glands. Its production greatly influences the sympathetic nervous system (for example, it increases during states of fear and anger). It stimulates physical activity and causes blood vessels to constrict. That is why, in tense emotional states, blood circulation to the extremities (such as the hands, feet, scalp) is diminished. Adrenaline also affects carbohydrate metabolism.

The adrenal glands are so important that a deficiency of their secretion is incompatible with life itself. To revitalize these glands is to improve the entire circulatory system and to recharge tissue cells.

The ovaries
These two almond-shaped glands, located one on either side of the uterus, produce the ovarian hormones *oestrogen* and *progesterone.* The production of these hormones is controlled by the anterior lobe of the pituitary gland.

The ovarian hormones, apart from their effects on the development of secondary sex characteristics, also influence metabolism.

The testes
Located in the scrotum, the testes or male sex glands produce *testosterone*, which is believed to influence the health and youthfulness of the tissues. They also have some effect on metabolism.

Both women and men secrete male and female hormones, each sex normally producing more of the one and less of the other as befits it.

The production of both these types of hormones must remain in harmonious balance, allowing for slight variations. Otherwise, undesirable side-effects appear (such as pattern baldness in women whose male hormone level rises, and excessive dandruff which has been linked with baldness).

An excess of the male hormone has been linked to the thinning of the fatty subsurface layer of the scalp, the function of which is partly to protect the scalp from undue compression by scalp and facial muscle tension.

The pancreas
Located, roughly, below the stomach, the pancreas is about 17.5cm (7 inches) long.

The gland has two functions: to secrete a very important digestive fluid — *pancreatic juice,* which contains digestive ferments that act on carbohydrates, fats and proteins, and to secrete the hormone *insulin* which plays a vital role in carbohydrate metabolism.

Connection with the nervous system

The endocrine glands are closely connected, functionally, with the nervous system. According to Dr Brena, the hormones are, in their intimate essence, further manifestations of electrochemical energy condensed inside the cells and tissues of the human body. He cites, as an example, the hormone adrenaline, which is formed by the adrenal glands as well as condensed at the end of sympathetic nerve fibres.

As I remarked at the beginning of this chapter, the endocrine system affects everything we do and influences our very existence. But all our systems are intimately interdependent, and the functioning of one will inevitably have a bearing on that of the others. If our endocrine glands are working harmoniously, there is no shortage or surplus of a particular hormone.

And this brings me to the theory that common baldness — the type that affects millions of people nowadays — is due to an overproduction of male hormones.

Male hormones and common baldness

The relationship between baldness and hormone secretion has been demonstrated by experiments performed by Dr J. B. Hamilton, an acknowledged expert on this topic. Using eunuchs as subjects, Dr Hamilton observed that there was immediate hair loss and a tendency to baldness when they were injected with male hormones. When the hormone injections were discontinued, however, the eunuchs' normal hair growth resumed.

As mentioned before, however, the normal functioning of all the endocrine glands is influenced by the anterior lobe of the pituitary or master gland. It is not inconceivable, therefore (in fact it is decidedly possible) that suboptimal functioning of this master gland would effect a similar lack of the male sex glands and result in an aberration of their hormone production and its balance with other hormones within the system. When the pituitary functions optimally, chances are that all the other glands and their secretion will be in harmonious equilibrium.

A dysfunction of the hormonal system, which upsets the functioning of other systems, may interfere with normal hair regeneration or with the cell-building phase of the body's metabolism. This, in turn, would influence the health and maintenance of the hair. In fact, endocrinologists have demonstrated distinct relationships between glandular disturbances and the growth of the hair.

In Chapter 9, I give exercises designed to stimulate the normal functioning of the pituitary and thyroid glands which influence the body's metabolic processes. With faithful practice and with patience, there is good reason to believe that these exercises may contribute to the harmony of the endocrine glands, so that any existing imbalance may possibly be corrected. With this in mind, and with the awareness, too, that there is usually no single cause for progressive hair loss but rather a combination of factors, I hope that optimism and perseverance will triumph over fatalism. As Dr Lubowe points out in his book, there are now too many known reasons for baldness and too many ways of coping with it to justify any other initial attitude but marked optimism.

Hormone preparations

One may well ask if the use of hormone preparations, either taken internally or applied externally, could not help to reactivate hair growth.

In the past few decades, scientists in various countries have tried this approach with such little success that their attempts, according to nutrition expert Dr Paavo Airola, were quietly abandoned. Moreover, whatever minute success there may have been was totally obliterated by the many undesirable side-effects these hormone treatments produced. For example, the administration of the female sex hormone oestrogen, to compensate for the overproduction of male sex hormones, has been known to have a feminizing effect on men (for example, producing breast enlargement), to inhibit the desire for sex and to reduce virility. Given a choice, which man would wish to lose his virility rather than his hair?

Oestrogen therapy has also been associated with abnormal blood clotting, inflammation of the veins and strokes.

In women, hormonal preparations may produce hair where it is least desired — on the face.

Instead of attempting to restore hormonal balance through the external or internal use of synthetic hormones, then, why not take the natural approach? Change your dietary habits so that they are more in keeping with a regime that provides the hair-strengthening substances your hair needs for vibrant health. Devote a portion of each day to exercises that will stimulate your glands beneficially and effect an improvement in the growth and quality of your hair. Incorporate into your life natural relaxation techniques to reduce facial and scalp tension, which impedes a rich blood flow to the hair's manufacturing plant (see Chapter 10). Determine to apply sound hair hygiene principles to keep your scalp free of particles that clog its pores (Chapter 12). You will find the above programme of long-term benefit not only to your hair and scalp but to your whole person as well.

9.

ESSENTIAL EXERCISES FOR HEALTHY HAIR GROWTH

Why exercise?

The exercises to follow are very special. They have been selected because of their amazing effects on the blood circulation, on the endocrine glands and on the nervous system.

We know that every single cell of the body depends on an adequate supply of blood for its nourishment, health and regeneration. This is no less true of the cells of the hair and scalp than it is of tissue anywhere else in the body. In fact, tissues at the extremities of the body (the *periphery*) often manifest signs of deficient circulation when the blood supply it receives is poor. This can happen, and often does, as a result of the difficulty the blood encounters as it circulates upward.

When the blood has to travel 'uphill', as in the case of the scalp circulation, it has to contend with the forces of gravity and, not infrequently, it reaches its destination impoverished.

If the peripheral (at the periphery) circulation is defective, the tissues beneath the scalp do not receive the nourishment they require to enable the hair factory located there (the hair bulbs and papillae) to produce as it should. Hair manufacture then falls. The blood, remember, is the life force of every body cell, carrying to it hormones, minerals, vitamins and other elements essential for the ongoing process of hair replacement.

We know, too, that the secretions of the endocrine glands influence the functioning of all the other systems of the body. Every organ, every cell, is under endocrine gland control. And the anterior lobe of the master gland — the pituitary — affects the status of the rest of the organism. The thyroid gland, too, influences the process of life by which tissue cells are destroyed and renewed (metabolism). The adrenal glands, as well, have a pervasive effect on the entire system. If these glands languish or are overactive, the nutrition and performance of every body cell will be affected accordingly.

We are aware, moreover, that the nervous system is intimately connected with the endocrine system. And so, whatever has a bearing on it will inevitably have repercussions on hormone production as well.

So, as has been pointed out before, all the body's systems are interdependent and work together, either for good or indeed for ill.

Preparing for the exercises

1. *Check with your doctor.* Obtain his or her permission to practise the exercises.
2. Practise regularly — better ten minutes six days a week than one hour once a week.
3. Try to exercise at the same time each day to establish what may be a new habit. Get up twenty minutes earlier in the morning than you have been used to doing. This will allow you ample time for your essential exercises. The effort will pay marvellous dividends. Are not ten minutes a day worth the prospect of improved hair growth and decelerating hair loss?
4. Empty your bladder; wear loose clothing; be comfortable. For maximum safety, remove sharp objects from your person (such as hairpins, pen, nail-file).
5. It is best to practise on an empty stomach, or at least not immediately after eating.
6. Always warm up first to avoid muscular pulls and strains.
7. Practise on a padded surface (such as a carpet or folded blankets on the floor; this padded surface will be referred to, from now on, as the 'mat').
8. When you first begin to do the exercises, you may practise each one two or three times, with a short rest period in between. As you are able to hold each position for a longer time, however, you need do each exercise once only — it is the holding period that produces the overall benefits.

The exercises have been arranged in a special sequence.

For best results, stick to this sequence as closely as possible.

Warm-ups

Neck warm-ups
1. Sit naturally erect on your mat. Rest your hands quietly on your lap. Breathe evenly. You may close your eyes or keep them open.
2. Imagine a large figure-eight, lying on its side, in front of you. Trace its outline with your nose or forehead or whole face. Try to keep your shoulders still as you do these head movements. Repeat the movements several times, in a smooth and connected manner. Do them slowly. Rest.
3. Repeat step 2 in the opposite direction, several times. Rest.

Note: Apart from its warm-up value, these head movements are excellent for reducing tension accumulated in the neck, and for encouraging a rich blood supply toward the scalp.

Shoulder warm-ups
1. Sit naturally erect on your mat. Rest your hands quietly at your sides. Breathe evenly.
2. Keeping your head still, rotate your shoulders smoothly, several times, in a front-to-back motion. Exercise slowly. Rest.
3. Repeat step 2 in a back-to-front motion. Rest.

Leg warm-ups
1. Sit naturally erect on your mat, legs stretched out in front.
2. Fold the legs inward, bringing the soles of the feet together.
3. Put your hands around the feet and pull them closer to the body. Maintain your upright position. Breathe naturally.
4. With a little upward pull on the feet, begin to flap the knees down and up, in smooth succession, like the wings of a butterfly.
   In time, you will be able to do as many as 100 flaps in about a minute.
5. To ease yourself out of this position, put your hands on the mat behind you, fingers pointing backward. Lean back slightly. Stretch out your legs. Rest.

All-body warm-up (rock-and-roll)
1. Sit on your mat. Bend your legs and place the soles of the feet on the mat, close to the bottom.
2. Pass your arms *under* the bent knees and hug your thighs. Curve your back to assume as rounded a position as possible. Tuck your head down.
3. Roll onto your back; kick backward.
4. Kick forward to come up again, but do not land heavily on your heels as this will jar your spine.
5. Repeat steps 3 and 4, several times in smooth succession, to massage and warm up your spine and spinal muscles and to stimulate the blood circulation.
6. Sit or lie down and relax.

You are now ready for the special sequence of hair regenerating exercises.

The headstand

Description
This is a position of perfect upside-down balance, in which the inverted body rests on a base in the form of an equilateral triangle. This triangle is formed by the head and the forearms.

Benefits
Because the blood circulation is not going 'uphill', as it usually does, a richer than usual blood supply reaches the upper body, particularly the head and scalp. You might say that these parts receive a sort of natural 'blood transfusion'.

Dr Paavo Airola writes (in *Stop Hair Loss*) that many persons have reported a better hair growth, and even new hair in previously bald areas, after practising the headstand regularly for a few months. He further comments that the regular performance of the headstand, in his opinion, is the single most important thing you can do to prevent hair loss and improve the health of your hair!

Modern medicine sometimes attempts to achieve such natural 'blood transfusions' by raising the legs of persons in what is called *Trendelenburg position*.

Because the pituitary gland is located in the head, it is beneficially stimulated by the improved blood supply to this area. And since it is the master gland, controlling all the other glands in the body's endocrine system, all these glands benefit in turn.

The discharge of blood from lower to upper body, effected by the headstand, is advantageous to the kidneys, stomach, intestines and sex glands. Because of this, the elimination of waste is enhanced, keeping the blood clean; digestion and absorption of food are improved, thus enriching the nutrition of all cells, especially those of the hair and scalp; sex hormone production is normalized for a more harmonious balance of the male and female hormones in the system.

The upside-down position has also been known to help turn grey hair to its original colour.

Caution: Persons suffering from any form of heart disease, high blood pressure and other circulatory problems as well as respiratory (breathing) disorders should *not* attempt this exercise.

Suggestions

When learning the headstand, ask someone to read the instructions, step by step, so that you can concentrate fully on the various stages involved.

Your helper can also alert you to any possibility of hurting yourself, although if you follow the instructions carefully, there should be no problem.

You may find it more comfortable to remove your ring(s) from your finger(s).

The headstand is such an important exercise for the scalp and hair that it should *not* be rushed. Several weeks spent on perfecting it, stage by stage, would be well worth while.

How to do it

Stage I

1. Sit on your heels. Let your toes point backward.
2. Lean forward and rest your elbows on the mat.
3. Adjust the distance between the elbows to measure the length of a forearm. This is done by swivelling the left forearm inward and fitting the space between thumb and forefinger snugly against the right upper arm, at the angle of the elbow. Do the same with the right forearm. From now on, *do not* shift the position of the elbows.

4. With the elbows firmly planted on the mat, swing the forearms forward, interlacing the fingers of one hand with those of the other.
5. Rest the top of your head on the mat between the palms; the back of the head is cradled against the hands.
6. Curl the toes so that they now point forward.
7. Press on the toes; lift and straighten the knees.

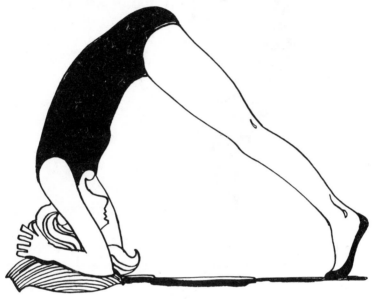

Figure 4   The Headstand — stage I

You are now in the head-low, hips-high position that marks the completion of stage I (Figure 4).

Don't be in a hurry to move on to stage II. Practise this part of the headstand each day until you are very comfortable with it. Breathe evenly while holding the position.

Hold the position for a few seconds to begin with. Increase the time until you can maintain the position for about a minute in absolute comfort.

In reverse motion, *very slowly,* come out of your position. Rest, sitting on your heels for a minute or two, before getting up.

You are now ready for stage II of the headstand.

Stage II

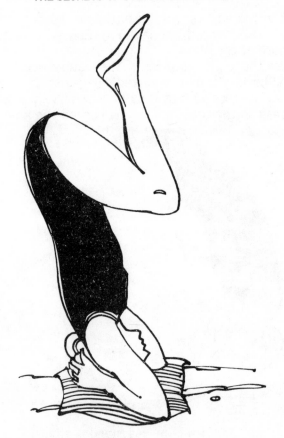

Figure 5   The Headstand — stage II

8. From the position described in step 7, walk on tiptoe toward your head until you feel almost as if the toes lift off the mat of their own accord. Bend the legs at the knees so that the toes point backward. The bent knees are close to the chest (Figure 5).

    This ends stage II of the headstand.

Practise holding this position, each day, until you're confident and ready for stage III.

Maintain the position for a few seconds to begin with, and work up to about a minute. Breathe evenly. In reverse motion, *very slowly*, come out of your position. Rest, sitting on your heels for a minute or two, before getting up.

You are now ready for stage III of the headstand.

Stage III

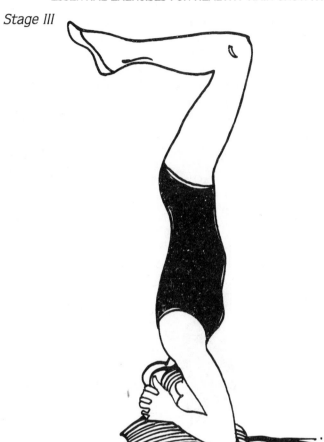

Figure 6 The Headstand — stage III

9. From the position described in step 8, straighten the hip joints so that the knees point upward and the heels point downward at the back (Figure 6).

Practise holding this position daily for an increasing length of time, as described previously. Breathe evenly. Slowly come out of the position, as outlined in the foregoing paragraphs.

Now proceed to the final stage of the headstand.

Stage IV

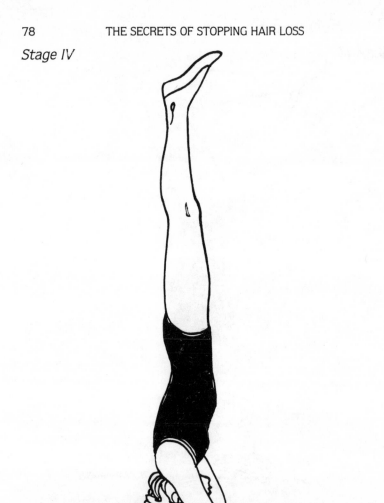

Figure 7   The Headstand completed

10. From the position described in step 9, straighten your knee joints until your feet point upward and your body is perfectly aligned (Figure 7).

Hold the position for a few seconds to begin with, increasing the time until you can effortlessly maintain it for about five minutes. Breathe evenly.

Coming out of the position

Always come out of the headstand position *very slowly*, in stages (corresponding to the stages described for going into position), until you are in the position described in step 5 of stage I.

Make fists; rest one on the other; rest your head on the fists for about a minute. Sit on your heels and rest. Slowly get up.

Comments on this exercise

Although seemingly difficult, the headstand can be mastered by anyone in reasonably good health (with your doctor's consent, of course).

It permits excellent relaxation of all muscles, since the axis of gravity from the barycentre (the prefix 'bary' indicates 'heavy') of the body drops exactly in the supporting triangle which forms the base of the headstand position.

Practise the headstand as a relaxation exercise, for a quick surge of fresh energy after a fatiguing day.

The shoulderstand

Whereas the headstand may be considered the king of all the exercises with the potential for improving hair growth, the shoulderstand may rightly be called the queen of exercises.

Description

This is another head-low, hips-high body position that summons the aid of gravitational forces. The all-body-reverse posture enables the blood to circulate more easily to the upper torso, enriching the tissues in that area with healthful nutrients.

Benefits

The health-giving benefits of the shoulderstand are the result of a two-fold mechanism: stretching and contraction of three groups of muscles. These are the back muscles, which are stretched, the abdominal muscles, which are contracted, and the muscles at the front of the neck, which are also contracted.

The organs within the trunk are revitalized: stomach, intestines, liver, pancreas, spleen, bladder and reproductive organs, bringing about improvement in digestive, metabolic and endocrine processes.

In stage II of this exercise, the pressure on the thyroid gland (created by the contraction of muscles at the front of the neck) and an increased blood supply to this area enhance thyroid function. Since the thyroid gland controls the entire metabolic process of the body, all tissues and all cells benefit.

This position of inverted balance has also been known to cause grey hair to recapture its original colour.

Caution: Persons suffering from heart disease, high blood pressure or other circulatory disorder, or from respiratory abnormalities should not practise this exercise without a doctor's consent.

Suggestions
A wall or other sturdy prop may be used as an aid to help you to get into position when you first attempt this exercise.

How to do it

Stage I

1. Lie on your back on your mat. Knees are bent; soles of the feet are flat on the mat; arms are close to the sides of the torso.
2. Bring the bent knees to the chest.
3. Straighten the legs so that the toes point upward.
4. Kick backward, simultaneously with both feet, until the hips are off the mat; support the hips with the hands — thumbs are in front (Figure 8). The weight of the lower body is borne by the palms, elbows, neck and back of the head, the elbows acting as a sort of fulcrum.

   Hold this position, breathing evenly, for a few seconds to begin with, working up to several minutes as you become more adept.

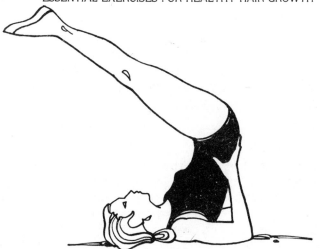

Figure 8   The Shoulderstand — stage I

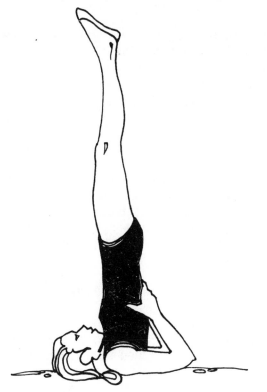

Figure 9   The Full Shoulderstand

To come out of position
Put the arms down beside the body; keep the head firmly pressed to the mat as you lower the hips; bend the knees; lower the feet to the floor; stretch out and rest.

When you can confidently hold the position described in step 4 for several minutes, proceed to stage II.

Stage II

5. Follow steps 2 to 4 of the shoulderstand, previously outlined.
6. Gradually move your hands, one at a time, from your hips toward your upper back, until your body is in as vertical a position as you can manage with complete comfort (Figure 9). Your chin, in the stage II position, should be in contact with your chest and your body as relaxed as possible.

Hold the position for a few seconds to begin with, working up to five minutes as you become more familiar with it. Breathe as naturally as possible.

To come out of the position
Tip the feet backward slightly and rest your arms beside your body. Keep your chin up and your head pressed to the mat as you slowly lower your hips to the mat; bend your knees; lower your feet to the mat; stretch out and relax.

Comments on the shoulderstand
If you have conscientiously tried the headstand and still cannot achieve it, concentrate on perfecting the shoulderstand. Its benefits are almost the same.

Use the shoulderstand as a relaxation exercise — for a quick 'pick-me-up' after a hard day.

The backstretch

Description
In this position, which is a logical sequel to the shoulderstand, the back muscles are stretched and the abdominal and front neck muscles are contracted to a greater extent than they are in the shoulderstand.

The body is not inverted, however, but folded over on itself.

Benefits

The benefits of the backstretch are as for the shoulderstand. In addition, because of a natural traction on the spine, any pinched nerves are freed, with consequent improvement in the functioning of the nervous system. Moreover, circulation to the spinal cord is accelerated.

Since the nervous and endocrine systems are closely interdependent, the latter profits as well, and both systems transmit their benefits to the cells of the hair and scalp.

As the position is held, with rhythmic breathing, the muscles at the back of the head and neck receive a gentle but very therapeutic massage. This stimulates the blood circulation to the scalp for the general health of the hair.

Caution: The same cautions for the shoulderstand apply here. Care, too, should be taken if any herniae are present (especially a hernia (protrusion) of the navel).

Suggestions

If your feet cannot reach the mat behind you at first, you may place a chair, stool or pile of cushions for the toes to touch, so as to get some idea of your progress.

How to do it

1. Begin as for the shoulderstand: lie on your back; knees bent; soles of the feet flat on the mat; arms straight and close beside the body.
2. Bring the bent knees to the chest.
3. Straighten the legs so that the feet point upward.
4. Kick backward, simultaneously with both feet, until the hips are off the mat. Keep the arms and hands where they are.
5. Keep pushing the feet backward; let the weight of the legs bear the feet toward the mat (or prop) behind you, reaching as far as they comfortably can (Figure 10).

Hold this position for a few seconds to begin with, working up to several minutes as you become more supple and comfortable in the posture. Breathe as naturally as you can.

To come out of the position

Slowly roll the spine onto the mat until the hips are down —

pressing the arms and hands firmly to the mat will help you do this with control. Keep the head firm on the mat.

Bend your knees; lower your feet to the mat; stretch out and relax.

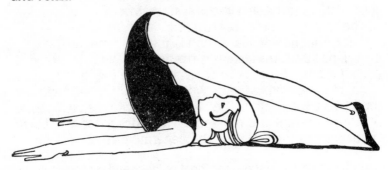

Figure 10   The Backstretch

Comments on the backstretch
If your feet do not immediately reach the mat behind you (or even your prop), do not despair. As the spine loses its initial stiffness, you will achieve your goal.

The backbend

Description
The backbend is a logical counterposition to the backstretch, providing a stretching of the abdominal and front neck muscles and a contraction of the back muscles.

Benefits
The thyroid gland, located in the neck, benefits from the therapeutic stretching of the throat. Because of thyroid influence on the body's entire metabolism, all processes profit.

The stretching of the whole front of the body is beneficial to other endocrine glands as well (for example, the sex glands). Because the rib-cage is well expanded, the lungs can be better ventilated, increasing the oxygen available to every body cell.

The contraction of the back muscles brings about a therapeutic massage of the adrenal glands, helping to enhance their function and their far-reaching effects on other body processes. The spinal muscles, too, benefit from this massage, as does the spinal circulation, thereby benefiting the whole nervous system.

Caution: This exercise is best avoided if herniae are present.

How to do it

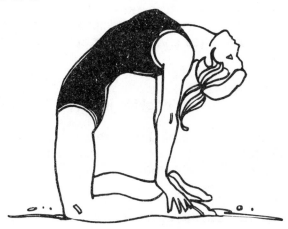

Figure 11   The Backbend

1. Kneel on your mat.
2. Lean back carefully and rest your left hand on your left heel.
3. Rest your right hand on your right heel.
4. Bracing hands on heels to steady yourself, *slowly and carefully* lean your head back; push the chest and hips upward to fully stretch the whole front of the body (Figure 11).

Hold your position for a few seconds, breathing as deeply and as evenly as possible. In time, hold your position for two or three minutes.

To come out of the position
Carefully bring your head up and slowly ease yourself into your beginning position. Sit on your heels and rest.

Advanced variation
To increase the stretch to the entire front of the body, place the hands on the floor behind the respective feet.

Easy variation
If you find the basic backbend difficult to do, try this simpler version:

1. Sit on the heels; toes point backward.
2. Lean back and place your hands on the mat behind the respective feet; fingers point backward.
3. Carefully tilt the head back; aim the front of the body upward as you slowly lift the hips from the heels.
4. Hold the position as long as you comfortably can, breathing steadily.

    Come out of the position, carefully, in reverse. Rest.

The folded leaf

In this exercise, a crouching posture is assumed, much like that adopted by some children during sleep or by certain religions to symbolize worship.

Benefits

The back muscles and spine are well stretched, and this enhances the spinal circulation and health of the spinal nerves. The entire nervous system shares this profit and this includes, of course, the nerve supply to the scalp.

    The head-low position affords the scalp and hair a richer than usual supply of blood, bringing to the cells in this area vital nutrients to help them to thrive and regenerate.

    While the position is being held, rhythmic breathing effects a beneficial massage to all glands, organs, blood vessels and other structures within the body, stimulating them to improved functioning, for the ultimate benefit of every cell from head to toe.

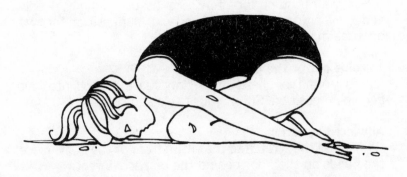

Figure 12 The Folded Leaf

Caution: Those persons suffering from high blood pressure should first check with their physician before practising this exercise.

How to do it

1. Sit on your heels; legs are together.
2. Lean forward and rest your forehead on the mat near the knees.
3. Rest the arms alongside the body, close to the legs; palms are upturned (Figure 12).

Hold this position for a few seconds to begin with, breathing evenly. In time, hold the posture for several minutes.

Variation
You may, if it is more comfortable, turn your head to one side for half of the holding period and to the other side for the rest of it.

To come out of the position
Simply raise first your head, then your torso and sit on your heels and rest.

Comment on the folded leaf posture
This is an excellent position in which to rest after a tiring day, and may be added to your repertory of relaxation techniques.

The spinal twist

This is perhaps the best exercise that gives maximum torsion (twisting) of the spine, with complete safety.

Benefits
The rotation of the spine effects a stimulating massage on the myriad nerves branching off the spinal cord. The result: the whole body and all the structures within it are revitalized.

The spinal rotation also massages the lower back muscles, benefiting in particular the adrenal glands which, as we now know, influence many body processes. According to Dr Steven Brena, to revitalize the adrenals is to improve the whole circulatory system and to 'recharge' all cellular 'electric batteries'.

The kidneys, too, benefit in their function of eliminating wastes from the system.

How to do it

1. Sit on the mat with your legs stretched out in front of you.
2. Bend the *left* leg at the knee; place the *left* foot beside the *outer right* knee.
3. Smoothly swivel your upper body to the *left*. Place both hands on the mat on the left *side*. Turn your head to look over your *left* shoulder (Figure 13).
4. Hold this position for a few seconds, breathing as regularly as you can. As you progress, hold it for a longer period.
5. Slowly untwist your body; stretch out your leg; rest.
6. Repeat steps 2 to 5, this time going in the other direction: substitute the word 'left' for 'right', and vice versa.

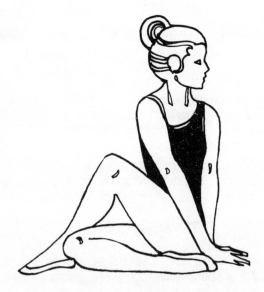

Figure 13   The Spinal Twist

10.
TENSION AND HAIR LOSS

Tension

Let no one tell you that tension does not have undesirable effects on the health of the hair and scalp. I am not referring to the basal tension in all muscles, without which we would collapse into a heap. Nor do I mean the tension of muscles at rest. Rather, I allude to the unnecessary build-up of tension of which so many of us are not even aware.

Here is an example. Say you want to write a letter. You need to tighten your fingers around the pen and, to some extent, tense arm and hand muscles. If not, the pen would slip from your fingers. So you exert only the required amount of tension to complete the job of letter-writing.

But suppose you are stuck for your next sentence. You bite on the top of the pen; you clench your teeth; you furrow your brow as you rack your brain for the right idea and words. These muscular overcontractions are absolutely unnecessary for either the finding of the right phrases or for writing them. They represent a waste of muscular energy and they take their toll on your health, in due course.

When we engage in such practices, we build up tension, which usually lodges in favoured areas: the face (particularly the jaws), the back of the neck, the shoulders. The tightened muscles exert undue pressure on adjacent structures (such as blood vessels and glands). The blood supply to these parts is impaired and the tissue it feeds becomes undernourished. It fails to thrive as nature intended. The glands either overproduce or underproduce. Their delicate balance is upset, and the whole body suffers.

This state of affairs exists regardless of whether the

overtense muscles are on the feet or indeed at the other end of the body — the face and head. Indeed, dentists will affirm that most of their clients have tight facial muscles.

If you look back at Chapter 3 (p. 29), you will note that the occipito-frontalis muscle runs from above the eyebrows, across the top of the head to the back of the skull. When you furrow your brow, it tightens this muscle; it draws the scalp forward. It is as if there were a drawstring around your scalp and when you frown, the drawstring tightens around the head. And any superficial observation of most adults would suggest that this wrinkling of the brow is not uncommon practice — the horizontal lines on the forehead are testimony enough.

The muscles of facial expression, too, are subject to much tension as we smile when we would rather not, either as a defence mechanism or to put up a front. Researchers say that habitual overcontraction of these muscles constrict the blood vessels of the scalp and impair nourishment to the hair. The situation is aggravated if these contractions occur suddenly and with force.

Review, too, the blood supply to the face and scalp (also in Chapter 3, p. 27) and you will appreciate that habits like clenching the teeth, biting on objects (such as the stem of a pipe or top of a pen or pencil), frowning, habitual gum-chewing and hunching of the shoulders, rather than maintaining an erect posture, will compress blood vessels in this area, of which there is a profusion.

And what about the hair muscles themselves — the erector pili or arrectores pilorum muscles (see also Chapter 3)? Anything that causes undue muscle tension will affect these hair muscles. They will pull on the hair and cause them literally to stand up. Over a long period of time (under conditions of long-term stress), this contraction of the arrectores pilorum, with its resulting constriction of adjacent blood vessels, will reduce the supply of oxygen and other nutrients to the hair. Abnormal hair fall will occur.

As far back as 1903, Dr Moritz Schein suggested that scalp tension was the cause of common or pattern-type baldness in humans. He had reason to believe that contraction of the scalp muscles reduced the supply of blood and lymph circulating in that area by compressing the skin and connective tissues.

Although Dr Schein thought that this compression was due

to an inherited shape of skull, the principle must surely apply to anything that produces a like constriction, namely, habitual facial and scalp tension resulting from, say, nervous facial expressions and other such bad habits.

Along similar lines are supporting theories by other researchers. Around the 1960s, Pohl-Pincus, a histologist (one who studies the microscopic structure of tissue) found tight compression of tissue in bald scalps of men. By contrast, scalp tissues were looser and thicker in women and children. (Women, by the way, usually have smaller, flatter heads than men, a shape that is thought to help protect them from this restricted blood supply to the scalp. This, however, seems to be changing — see 'Stress and hair loss' later in this chapter.)

As if in confirmation, Dr Irwin I. Lubowe has offered from his own clinical practice the observation that women who consulted him because of pattern-type baldness usually have very tight scalps and a very thin layer of fat and subcutaneous (under the skin) tissues.

In an interesting experiment carried out by a Howard University anatomist, Dr M. Wharton Young, elliptical pieces of scalp were removed from monkeys. The skin edges were then stitched together to produce a tighter scalp. The result: a persistent baldness resembling that occurring in humans.

In yet another study, Dr Young found that scalp tension causes thinning of the scalp underpadding, which interferes with the circulation of the hairs and results in hair loss. Examining X-rays of scalps well-endowed with hair, he noted that this tissue underpadding was twice the thickness of that under the forehead or under a scalp devoid of hair.

Pursuing the connection between hair loss and tension, two University of Chicago psychiatrists, Dr Thomas A. Szasz and Dr Alan M. Robertson spent much time studying baldness in relation to nervous causes. They found evidence to support the observation that facial tension (for instance, in the form of a habitual forced grin or smile) or frequent explosive laughter produced considerable scalp tension leading to compression of structures vital to the flourishing of the hair.

These are but a handful of the findings of intelligent, dedicated researchers in the field of hair growth and hair loss. Scientific literature abounds with other persuasive evidence of the tension-baldness connection, and the consensus of the most knowledgeable experts is that the functions primarily involved in hair growth are those of the circulatory and glandular systems, and that both can be influenced!

Stress and hair loss

As noted previously in this book, there is now no question that the incidence of abnormal hair loss among men and women has increased in the last few decades. Hair experts believe that the most outstanding reason for this is stress in the various forms it takes in present-day living. And stress — the body's reaction to demands made upon it — produces tension.

Encouragingly, though, the experts say that in so far as hair loss is caused by stress, it is treatable.

Here are some of the things stress does to your hair and its related structures:

1. It affects the hair follicles, muscles, nerves and blood vessels; by constricting the tiny blood vessels — the capillaries — feeding the hair follicles, it limits the amount of oxygen and other nutrients reaching the hair.
2. Stress causes excessive sweating.
3. Sweat combined with airborne pollutants makes the scalp and hair dirtier than usual.
4. I have already explained how tension affects the hair muscles, and since stress causes increased tension, it obviously adversely influences the blood supply reaching the hair because it constricts the blood vessels.
5. Stress causes increased secretion of the sebaceous, or oil-producing, glands and so contributes to dandruff formation.

The well-known British trichologist, Philip Kingsley, has remarked that stress is, without question, *the single most dangerous condition* that confronts the career woman (my emphasis). This is, he has added, because it is highly injurious to her hair and to the rest of her body as well.

In summary, then, as the tension of muscles mounts, the muscles lying under the scalp proportionately contract. This exerts extra pressure on the blood vessels located there; they constrict or become narrower. The blood flow is consequently slowed down or lessened. The nutrients the blood contains cannot satisfactorily reach the hair follicles. They languish, and the hair weakens. In time, it gives up its struggle for

therefore, is potentially disadvantageous to the wellbeing of the hair.

What can we do about tension?

The soundest, most enduring approach to this question of excessive tension, then, is a daily regimen of relaxation techniques which, in this busy era, would best be incorporated into daily schedules until they become almost second nature. These techniques, as well as the exercises in Chapter 9, must be practised regularly to be of true and lasting value.

With these considerations, I have purposely designed the techniques to follow so that they are uncomplicated, enjoyable and adaptable to location and circumstance (they can be done in a variety of places, sometimes with slight modification). Make them an integral part of your life, like eating and brushing your teeth and going to bed. Your hair will be infinitely grateful.

Relaxation techniques

Facial relaxation

Benefits
This facial relaxation technique brings a rich blood supply to the scalp and facial tissues. It helps you to acquire an awareness of facial tension, which restricts the blood flow to the hair manufacturing plant beneath the scalp. It enables you to reduce that tension and so encourage nutrients to the scalp to help to regenerate the hair cells.

How to do it

1. Sit on your heels; put your hands on your knees. (You may also do this exercise sitting elsewhere or standing naturally erect.)
2. Inhale steadily.
3. Exhale and stick out your tongue as far as possible; open your eyes as widely as you can; look your fiercest (Figure

14). Hold the pose as long as your exhalation lasts.
4. Inhale and relax all facial muscles; close your eyes; visualize all tension draining from face and scalp.

Repeat this exercise several times during the day.

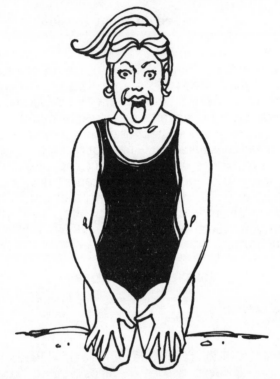

Figure 14   Facial Relaxation Exercise

Jaw relaxation

Benefits
Jaw tension is widespread. It has been linked to diminished blood circulation to the scalp and consequent hair loss. This exercise helps to establish an awareness of accumulating tension in the jaws. It enables you to eliminate that tension, consciously, before it creates undue pressure on nearby blood vessels. It helps to send a rich surge of health-giving blood to the hair cells.

How to do it

1. Sit or stand anywhere you find comfortable. Maintain an erect posture.
2. Voice, or silently mouth, the following sentence, exaggerating the vowels marked:

Pā māy wē all gō too?

Your recitation may sound (or feel) like this:

Pah may wee awl go too?

Practise this several times during the day, including when caught in traffic, in waiting rooms, or at bus stops if you can do so unobtrusively, or in the bathroom.

Neck relaxation

Benefits
The following techniques help to dissolve tensions that cling to the back of the neck and throat. They help to bathe that area with a rich supply of blood containing nutrients that feed the hair and scalp cells.

Because two major arteries run along the neck (they have branches that feed the face and scalp), any accumulated tension in these parts causes kinking of these important blood vessels and interferes in their work of enriching the scalp and hair. The neck relaxation technique helps to remove pressures from this vital source of life to the hair cells.

How to do it

1. Sit or stand naturally erect where there is no impediment to free head movement. Breathe naturally.
2. Inhale. Exhale and turn your head to look as far to the *right* as you comfortably can (Figure 15). Hold this position and breathe in, out and then in again.
3. Exhale and turn your head to look straight forward. Inhale.
4. Exhale and turn your head to look as far to the *left* as you comfortably can. Hold this position and breathe in, out and then in again.

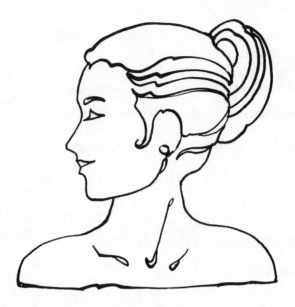

Figure 15   Neck Relaxation — first movement

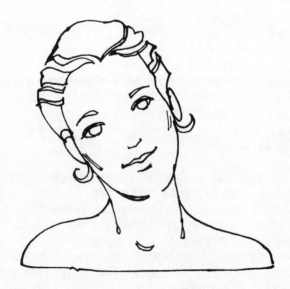

Figure 16   Neck Relaxation — second movement

5. Exhale and turn your head to look straight forward.
6. Repeat steps 2 to 5 a few times, slowly and in smooth succession. Rest.

Now proceed to:

7. Tilt your *right* ear toward your right shoulder, keeping the shoulder as steady as possible and moving only the head and neck (Figure 16).

Hold this position for a few seconds, breathing steadily.

8. Bring your head up again.
9. Repeat step 7 to the *left* (substitute the word 'left' for 'right').
10. Bring your head up again. Rest.

Apart from the foregoing, you may also practise the neck warm-ups described in Chapter 9, with similar benefit.

Please also refer to Chapter 13 where you will find instructions for correct scalp massage procedure (pp. 129-130).

Relaxation through breathing

You carry it with you everywhere. It is intimately connected with the way you feel. It is one of the handiest, most effective relaxation tools at your disposal — your breath. Use it to help you eliminate built-up tension and relax.

Rhythmic breathing
1. Sit or stand with your spine well aligned. (You can also practise this technique lying.) Relax your jaws by unclenching your teeth. Relax your hands and any other parts of your body that are obviously tense. If convenient, close your eyes.
2. Inhale slowly, smoothly and as deeply as you can without the least strain. *Do not* hold the breath.
3. Exhale slowly, smoothly and as thoroughly as possible, to expel every trace of stale air from your lungs.
4. Repeat steps 2 and 3, in smooth succession, for at least a minute. In time, work up to five minutes of rhythmic breathing.

Visualization

To enhance the effects of your rhythmic breathing exercise, visualize, as you inhale, a rich intake of oxygen entering your lungs and bloodstream and passing to every body cell, including your hair cells, to revitalize them.

As you exhale, imagine waste matter from all the cells and tissues and blood drifting away with the expelled carbon dioxide.

Visualization is an ancient technique. It can be a powerful ally. It has long been used in the USSR and elsewhere to train athletes to excel in their chosen fields. It has been employed as an adjunct to other therapies to help bring about a remission in cancer patients whose prognosis was hopeless. It can be used in any endeavour to reinforce the effectiveness of other treatments. Make use of it. You may be amazed at what can come about through visualization.

General relaxation

Take between ten and twenty minutes each day to practise the following relaxation technique which is being recommended by many enlightened doctors to their patients to counteract the deleterious effects of accumulated tension.

1. Sit comfortably in an armchair or recliner or lie down on a carpeted surface or bed or couch, in a face-upward position.
2. Separate your legs so as to discourage an accumulation of tension in the thighs and hips.
3. Shift the arms away from the sides of your body so as to discourage tension build-up in the upper arms and shoulders. Turn your palms upward.
4. Check for jaw tension: unclench the teeth. This helps with a freer flow of breath into and out of the lungs.
5. Close your eyes.
6. Shift your focus of attention to your breathing. Mentally observe the rhythmic rise and fall of your abdomen as air enters and leaves the body. As you begin to shed your tensions, the breath will become slower and more even. And as the breath becomes more regular and natural, it will enhance the relaxation of your whole being, so interdependent are body and breath. Spend about a

minute on this silent meditation upon your breath.

7. Now direct your attention to the feet. In your mind, say to the toes and feet: 'Toes, let go of your tightness; relax. Feet, let go of your tension; relax.' Concentrate only on the feet, isolating them, as it were, from the rest of your body. Spend several seconds on this part of the body, until you are aware that it is responding positively to your silent suggestions.

8. Now shift your focus of attention to your calf muscles. As you did with the feet, give to the calves positive mental suggestion to let go of tightness and to relax completely. When the calves respond and begin to relax, go on to the thighs.

9. As in steps 7 and 8, give positive mental suggestion to the powerful thigh muscles to let go of their tightness and to relax. When they respond favourably, do the same with all the other parts of your body, in turn. Do this systematically, remembering to cover:

- the buttock muscles
- the small of the back
- the shoulder-blades and upper back
- the abdomen
- the chest
- the fingers and palms
- the forearms
- the upper arms
- the shoulders
- the back of the neck
- the throat
- the tongue
- the jaws
- the lips
- the cheeks
- the eyes
- the eyelids
- the forehead and the scalp

10. Finally, direct your thoughts, once again, to your breathing and now apply the visualization technique:

Each time you inhale, visualize taking into the body a fresh supply of vital energy and positive things; and each time you exhale, imagine sending away from your system all frustrations, all fatigue and everything negative. With each exhalation, too, relax a little more; let yourself go totally; relax, relax, relax!

To come out of your deep relaxation

Don't rush! Make the transition from deep relaxation to activity slow, smooth and conscious. Wiggle fingers and toes. Yawn if you wish. Roll your head from side to side. Leisurely stretch the limbs — whatever your body dictates. Roll onto your side, knees bent, and use your arms and hands to help you into the sitting position (if you were lying).

Slowly stand up, stretch sensuously from top to toe and revel in the deliciously refreshed feeling you experience.

Anxiety and hair loss

Dr Irwin I. Lubowe has observed that as long as anxiety is present, no form of treatment, however effective under other conditions, is likely to work. The anxiety, he adds, will literally push out the hair from the scalp faster than the treatment can replace it! Something has got to give — either the anxiety or the hair; and chances are that anyone having a choice would choose to relinquish the former and hang on to the latter.

Experts agree that since increasing hair loss tends to generate anxiety and even fear, these emotions reinforce factors already contributing to the hair loss and a vicious circle is formed.

As the distress of these negative emotions increases, the tissues underlying the scalp tighten. This places pressure on the innumerable blood vessels located there; they constrict; their flow is impeded. With this blood-flow restriction, there is a corresponding diminution of life-giving nutrients to the hair cells. They starve, and die; the hair is shed.

Meditation can help

One of the most effective ways to deal with anxiety, obvious or concealed, is the daily practice of meditation. I have worked with doctors who have prescribed meditation twice daily, twenty minutes each session, in cases where an existing anxiety aggravated other ailments.

The physiological benefits of regular meditation are now well documented. Meditation helps to diminish tensions that interfere with the optimal functioning of the blood circulation, hormone production and balance, and with other vital body processes. Not even deep sleep or dream states can ease such strains in the same way.

During meditation, a physiologically unique state occurs. Oxygen consumption and carbon dioxide elimination decrease significantly; but the normal balance between the two is unchanged, signifying satisfactory blood circulation. The heart rate slows down, as does the breathing, denoting a state of deep rest which is highly beneficial to all cells. It gives them welcome respite from constant activity and helps in their regeneration. Skin resistance increases markedly — an index of deepening relaxation. The body's metabolic rate slackens by about 20 per cent, with a corresponding lowering of the blood pressure and lessening of strain on the heart. The lactate ion concentration in the blood, which is high in anxiety states, decreases by about 33 per cent. Electroencephalograph (EEG) recordings (of brain activity) show an unusual abundance of alpha waves, a sure sign that the brain is rested, yet superbly alert.

How to meditate
Set aside ten to twenty minutes once or twice a day, before a meal. A full stomach and the process of digestion interfere with the concentration required for proper meditation.

Arrange your affairs so as not to be interrupted during this time. Choose a quiet place for your practice.

Sit naturally erect. You may use a prop to support the spine and keep it well aligned.

Be at ease so that physical discomfort does not distract you from your meditation.

Close your eyes. Establish and maintain a steady, easy breathing rhythm that is the most natural for you.

Relax every part of your body as well as you can.

Inhale. *Exhale* and mentally say a predetermined word, such as 'peace', 'relax', 'tranquillity' or 'one'.

Continue this silent recitation of your chosen word, *always on the exhalation.*

At first, your thoughts will drift away often from your concentration on your word. Do not let this unsettle you. Coax your attention back to it. In time, this diversion will lessen. Persevere, but do not force anything, as this will generate tensions that defeat the purpose of the exercise.

After a while, you will feel a natural impulse to get up. Do not rush to do so. Make the transition from relative inactivity to routine activity slow and smooth. Open your eyes; stretch your limbs leisurely; increase the depth of your breathing. Slowly get up.

In the beginning, you may find that five minutes are all you can comfortably spend in actual meditation. This is fine. Try again later today or tomorrow. With regular practice, you should gradually increase your meditation period to twenty minutes at least once a day, preferably twice.

A very good book to read on this subject is *The Relaxation Response* by Herbert Benson.

11.
KEEPING THE BLOOD CLEAN

Africans and their diet

A British doctor named Denis Burkitt, who worked in Africa for two decades, has reported that in the African countries there is little evidence of blood circulatory problems like those affecting the inhabitants of affluent countries such as ours. His research, studies and findings persuasively suggest that it is because of their high-fibre diet.

Is it merely coincidence that Africans and citizens of Third World countries usually boast luxuriant heads of hair? In the light of the fact that hair needs a plentiful, unrestricted supply of clean, nutrient-rich blood to flourish, Dr Burkitt's findings would explain, in part, why the population of these countries are more happily hirsute than we are.

The African diet (like that in third world countries) offers a daily intake of about 40-60g (1 ½-2 oz) of fibre (indigestible carbohydrate), which is 2½ times the amount most of us consume each day. Moreover, even in cases where Africans show considerable atherosclerosis (clogging of arteries by fatty deposits), blood clots seem to break down more quickly than they do in the western population. The high-fibre content of the stool appears, somehow, connected with a low blood cholesterol level and the relative absence of conditions associated with an obstructed blood supply.

For a wealth of information on this topic, and for Dr Burkitt's findings in more detail, read *Eat Right — To Stay Healthy and Enjoy Life More.*

After food has been eaten, digested and absorbed, the residue is passed along to the large intestine, or colon, by peristalsis (the wave-like contraction of tubular organs, which pushes their contents onward). Here, it awaits expulsion.

In the colon, peristalsis is very slow. It usually takes between sixteen and twenty-four hours for the colon's contents to pass through its length in readiness for elimination.

Africans digest and excrete their food (this is known as 'transit time') three times faster than do Europeans and Americans. Transit time among Africans is twenty-four hours or less. Among Europeans and Americans, it is an average of three days!

For rural Africans, the weight of the stool is usually three times heavier than it is for westerners. Urban Africans who adopt western dietary habits soon fall prey to the blood circulatory ailments that plague us. Immigrants from African countries quickly manifest signs of hair loss as they readily incorporate our dietary and postural habits into their lifestyle.

Auto-intoxification

The delay in transit time of waste from the system sets up a vicious condition known as 'auto-intoxification'. Normally, the waste products of digestion are expelled or neutralized reasonably quickly. However, when these products remain in the colon longer than they should, a self-poisoning process occurs and reabsorption of toxins takes place. The poisons that should have been cast off are thrown back into the bloodstream and carried to the tissues, and every cell of the body, from toes to head, suffers the consequences. It is the very bloodstream that conveys vital nutrients to the scalp and hair that carries away the body's waste products.

Another vicious circle is then created. The lining of the entire alimentary canal, which includes the stomach and small intestine, becomes inflamed. Malassimilation of nutrients, malnutrition and cell deterioration are some of the results.

A rule of thumb, then, for healthy hair growth and hair regeneration, is that no food residues should remain in the colon longer than twenty-four hours. Evacuation of the bowel should take place *at least once a day*.

Constipation

When the diet is deficient in fibre (also called bulk, roughage or cellulose), there can be, and often is, difficulty in ridding the body of waste matter on a daily basis. A condition of simple constipation arises. Even if partial elimination is accomplished, some faecal matter (stool) remains and contributes to a self-poisoning process. Cumulative constipation follows if steps are not taken to correct this state of affairs. The colon becomes more and more sluggish and only the pressure of built-up waste pushes out some of its contents.

But faulty diet is not the only culprit responsible for constipation. Flabby abdominal muscles that lack tonus (tone or tonicity), a lax pelvic floor (lowest part of the torso) and a lazy respiratory diaphragm (the muscle forming the floor of the chest cavity and dome of the abdominal cavity) are equally culpable accomplices.

Fortunately, all the foregoing conditions can be remedied. All you need are the desire to correct them and the persistence in applying the suggested antidotes which follow in the form of a detoxification plan.

The detoxification plan

Increasing your fibre intake
In Chapter 4, I mentioned some natural sources of fibre and gave hints on how to incorporate them into your diet. Food consultants suggest blending a tablespoon or two of natural wheat bran (available at supermarkets and health food stores) into a glass of unsweetened fruit or vegetable juice and drinking it once a day.

Some people add bran to their breakfast cereal, cold or hot. Remember that, of all the natural food fibre sources the unrefined bran (outer layer) of the wheat kernel is by far the best.

Another way to enhance your dietary fibre intake is to eat potatoes with their skins and a generous helping of fresh, raw vegetables and fruits every day. Eat dried fruit, like figs and prunes, as often as you can.

Improving muscle tone
Because the mechanism of defaecation (stool evacuation) brings into play the muscles of the abdomen, pelvic floor and respiratory diaphragm, all exercises that improve the tone and function of these structures are of value in combating constipation.

I have selected, and now offer you, what I consider to be the three best of such exercises. Practise them every day. Your general feeling of wellbeing will increase as your bloodstream becomes purer, and all the cells of your body more invigorated. Hair growth activity will revive as toxins are more thoroughly and regularly eliminated.

The abdominal lift

Caution: Do *not* practise this on a full stomach. The best time to do the abdominal lift is when the stomach is empty or near-empty, such as in the morning before breakfast, or at night three or four hours after dinner.

If you have high blood pressure, peptic ulcer (of the stomach or intestine) or any heart problem, omit this exercise. In any event, *check with your doctor* before you attempt the abdominal lift.

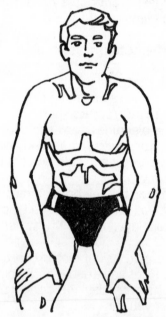

Figure 17   The Abdominal Lift

How to do it

1. Stand with your feet about 25cm (10 inches) apart.
2. Bend your knees and turn them slightly outward, as if preparing to sit.

3. Place your hands on the respective thighs. Keep the torso as erect as you comfortably can in this position.
4. Inhale. Now *exhale*.
5. With the *air still expelled*, briskly pull your abdominal muscles *inward*, as if to touch your spine with them, and *upward* toward your rib-cage (Figure 17).
6. Hold the abdominal contraction until you feel a strong impulse to inhale.
7. Inhale, straighten yourself and rest.

When you can perform the abdominal lift effectively and with ease, try this variation.

Variation
Follow steps 1 to 5 of the instructions for the basic exercise.

Hold the abdominal contraction for a second or two and, *with the breath still out*, briskly 'snap' the abdomen outward; pull it inward and upward. Repeat this inward-and-upward/ outward action five times in succession.

As you become adept at the technique, work up to twenty abdominal lifts per exhalation.

This variation provides a very effective massage of the colon to help stimulate peristalsis.

The bellows breath
Most of the time we breathe shallowly. Only our chest muscles come into play and then, only minimally. This makes for poor oxygenation (saturation with oxygen) of the tissues and an incompetent respiratory diaphragm.

Trained singers and public speakers are disciplined in the effective use of their diaphragm, which is considered the prime muscle of the exhalation phase of the breathing process. The diaphragm, too, as already mentioned, is intimately involved in the evacuation of the bowel. If the diaphragm is not strong and if it is not properly used, its function becomes impaired. Moreover, if the abdomen — which houses the diaphragm — is flabby and of poor tone, it would not have the required strength and elasticity to assist the diaphragm in its work of expulsion.

The bellows breath provides excellent training in the use and control of the diaphragm and abdominal muscles. Practised regularly, this breathing exercise will help to bring strength and efficiency to these important structures.

Caution: Check with your doctor before practising this dynamic breathing exercise. In any case, omit it if you have high blood pressure, a hernia or a heart problem.

At a hint of lightheadedness, immediately stop the exercise. Sit or lie quietly and rest before resuming activity.

1. Sit or stand with the spine well aligned. Put your fingers lightly against the midline of your abdomen, just below the ribs.
2. Inhale slowly, smoothly and deeply.
3. Briskly contract your abdomen (feel it tighten) to expel the air in your lungs forcefully. This is similar to the explosive action of sneezing.
4. Relax. The air will enter your lungs again without your help — a sort of involuntary inhalation.
5. You may relax your arms now that you have an idea of what is taking place.
6. For about a minute to begin with, repeat steps 2 to 4 in brisk, jerky succession: forceful exhalation followed by involuntary inhalation.

   As you become practised, you may increase the length of time you spend on this exercise.

Helpful hints
For best results, practise the bellows breath outdoors. When the oxygen content of the air is good the blood benefits and through it the hair cells. Without an adequate oxygen supply, cells languish.

Practise the bellows breath as part of your daily warm-up session, before starting your exercise routine. It will slightly increase your body temperature, cleanse your lungs and help you to concentrate better.

The knee presses

Caution: If you have high blood pressure, ask your doctor's permission to attempt this exercise.

How to do it

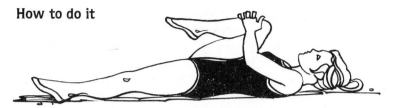

Figure 18   The Knee Press — using one leg

1. Lie on your mat. Legs are stretched out and arms are beside you. Breathe naturally.
2. Inhale. Exhale and bend the right knee. Bring it toward the chest. Clasp your hands around the knee (Figure 18).
3. Hold this position for several seconds, breathing normally.
4. On an exhalation, lower your arms and leg and rest. Repeat steps 2 to 4 three times.
5. Repeat steps 2 to 4 with the left leg, three times.
6. Now bend both knees, one at a time, and bring them to the chest. Hug them. Hold the position for as long as you are comfortable, breathing normally (Figure 19).
7. Relax the arms and legs.

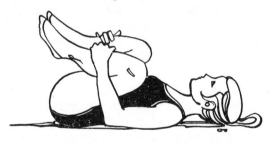

Figure 19   The Knee Press — using both legs

Squatting

In countries like China, Mexico, the West Indies, Vietnam and most in Africa, it is a not uncommon sight to see people squatting. They squat to chat informally, to eat, to wash clothes, to garden, or to await the homecoming of a family member.

We, by comparison, are a nation of chair-sitters, and this has made it difficult for us to assume, and to hold, a squatting posture, which is the position most mechanically suited to defaecation.

It is an interesting point that, in those countries where squatting is part of the way of life, constipation is the exception rather than the rule, and luxuriant heads of hair are commonplace and baldness a rare sight.

Granted, our society would frown upon bus-stop or sidewalk squatters, but surely no one would mind if we squatted to weed our garden, to watch television in the privacy of our home or to chat with a friend at the beach?

As we hold the squatting position and continue our rhythmic breathing, a gentle yet superbly stimulating massage of the intestines takes place. Peristalsis is promoted; elimination is enhanced and the bloodstream is detoxified to the ultimate benefit of every cell in the organism.

Let us look for ways to incorporate squatting into our life. (I usually squat in the bathtub to shampoo my hair and to shower. This is easy if the showerhead is attached to a hose.)

The following are hints to help to make this position as easy to do and to hold as nature intended.

Aids to squatting

1. You need supple ankles to squat for any length of time. Sit on a chair or stool or other comfortable prop. Stretch out your legs. Rotate your ankles ten times this way and ten times that way, slowly and smoothly. Rest.
2. Stand. Keep the feet firmly planted on the floor or mat or wherever you are.

    Bend the knees and ankles as if preparing to sit. Lower the body as far as you comfortably can.

    Straighten up. Repeat the up-and-down movements ten times. Rest.
3. Refer to Chapter 13. Practise the dog stretch exercise often (pp. 131-132).

How to squat

1. Stand tall. Breathe naturally.
2. Bend the legs and lower the body until the bottom comes close to the heels (Figure 20). You may either hug your knees or rest your arms at your sides.

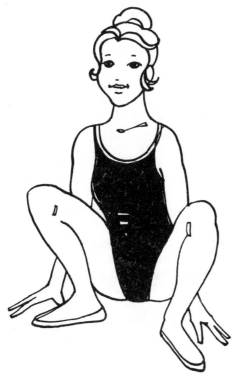

Figure 20   Squatting

Helpful hint
You may hold on to a table or other stable prop for support
when first learning to squat.

Other anti-constipation measures
Regularly practise the headstand, shoulderstand, backstretch,
backbend, the folded leaf and the spinal twist (see Chapter 9).

Commercial laxatives
Commercially prepared laxatives irritate the delicate lining of
the intestines. They interfere with digestion, and hamper
absorption.

Perhaps the most harmful of all laxatives are those with
a mineral oil base. Mineral oil is not a food; it cannot be
digested. About 60 per cent of mineral oil reaching the
intestine passes into the bloodstream. As it circulates

throughout the body, it attracts to itself, absorbs and holds captive the fat-soluble vitamins A, D, E and K. Later, it excretes them in the faeces (stool). In time, this may cause a vitamin deficiency.

For decades, the American Medical Association and medical journals have been warning doctors not to prescribe to patients laxatives containing mineral oil. And yet they continue to do so and patients persist in using these products.

Natural laxatives
Foods high in natural fibre provide natural laxative action. These have been mentioned in Chapter 4 and earlier in this chapter (p. 105).

The following makes an excellent natural laxative:

Mix well together: 15ml (1 tablespoon) each powdered mandrake, buckthorn bark, rhubarb root, fennel seed and calamus root, and 5 ml (1 teaspoon) aloes — all available from herbalists.

Put 1ml (a quarter-teaspoon) of the blended herbs in half a glass or less of cold water; stir well. Strain the liquid, if necessary, and drink it before going to bed at night.

An alternative is to mix together about 30g (1 oz) each of mandrake root, cascara sagrada bark, buckthorn bark, fennel seed and calamus root, and about 7g (¼ oz) aloes. Use as directed in the previous recipe.

You may follow your natural laxative drink with several sips of warm water to enhance the effects.

Another excellent natural laxative comes from the leaves of the peach tree. According to Jethro Kloss, author of *Back to Eden*, these leaves should be on hand in every home. Make a tea of them and sip the beverage slowly whenever the need arises.

Other aids to elimination
Take plenty of outdoor exercise such as brisk walking, bicycling, swimming, horseback riding, rowing, and so forth. Practise breathing deeply and rhythmically whenever you are in the fresh air to exercise the diaphragm and abdominal muscles.

Do not rush your visits to the toilet, but equally do not

postpone them. Make daily evacuation of the bowel a priority.

If constipation persists, you may have to resort to an occasional enema. Check first with your doctor, then try this natural enema solution.

Mix together equal portions of red raspberry leaves and wild cherry bark or leaves (or bayberry bark). These are available at herbalists.

Steep 5ml (1 heaped teaspoon) of the blend in 1.1l (2 pints) of hot water, as if you were brewing tea. Leave the mixture for ten to twenty minutes, strain and cool it to body temperature (approximately 98°F, or 37°C).

This enema solution disinfects the bowel to help rid it of putrefactive material. It stimulates it to improve peristalsis which helps to eliminate waste matter.

Recipe: Hi-fibre raw vegetable salad

¼ medium-size head green cabbage ⎫ grated or
1 large carrot, scrubbed, unpeeled ⎬ shredded (but
¼ small, peeled onion ⎭ not too finely)
2 radishes, trimmed, washed and chopped
1 handful alfalfa sprouts
30ml (2 tablespoons) unrefined oil (such as sunflower seed or safflower)
15ml (1 tablespoon) apple cider vinegar
A sprinkling of freshly ground peppercorns
A dash only of salt (optional)
125ml (½ cup) buttermilk or plain, unsweetened yogurt
5ml (1 teaspoon) raw or Demerara-style sugar

Mix well together the first five ingredients (the vegetables). Add the oil and again mix thoroughly. Add the vinegar, pepper, salt if you wish and sugar.

Again mix well. Finally, add the buttermilk or yogurt and stir well into the salad.

If not serving right away, cover and refrigerate.

This is my own version of American cole slaw. It is a decided favourite in my home. Do try it.

12.

A TREASURY OF
HAIR HYGIENE HINTS

Scalp hygiene

Scalp hygiene, emphasize authorities like Dr Irwin Lubowe, is the number-one prerequisite for anyone who wants to keep his or her hair and keep it healthy. Often, they say, proper hygiene practices faithfully carried out will be effective enough in controlling hair loss, even without other therapy. On the other hand, no course of treatment will bring about desired results without adherence to good hygiene habits.

Everything learned about the maintenance of hair suggests that the key elements of stimulation, cleansing and feeding are vital to hair growth and regeneration. These form the basis of good scalp and hair hygiene.

For hair to grow and thrive and renew itself, the scalp must be kept loose and its blood supply must be rich and unimpeded. Furthermore, the natural scalp secretions must be adequately produced and distributed. These requirements may be met admirably by pre-shampoo scalp conditioning, massage during shampoo (and in between shampoos) and by daily combing and brushing, provided that the proper tools and techniques are used.

Pre-shampoo conditioning

The scalp, like skin elsewhere in the body, provides us with a waterproof covering. But even the most glabrous (smooth) pate contains tiny openings (pores), as mentioned previously (p. 25). These miniscule conduits allow for some absorption of local applications, and although such topical treatments can never replace vital substances taken in systemically, they may nevertheless be used as adjuncts to enhance their value.

Many commercially prepared hair care products are potentially harmful to the hair and scalp. Some are too harsh and alkaline, upsetting the scalp's natural acid mantle or pH. The claims made on the labels or in the literature accompanying many of these products are far-fetched. It is the fingertip massage recommended during application of such commodities that provides the most benefit. Let the buyer beware!

Herbs for healthy hair

But herbal hair conditioners have been used for ages in the treatment of hair loss. Because they are natural, their absorption does not harm, but rather benefits, the scalp and the hair.

High-protein conditioner
Blend together, preferably in an electric blender:

    250ml (1 cup) skimmed milk
    1 egg yolk
    contents of 2 capsules wheat germ oil   )   available at
    15ml (1 tablespoon) fresh wheat germ   }   health food
    15ml (1 tablespoon) lecithin granules   {   stores
    15ml (1 tablespoon) natural wheat bran   )

Massage the mixture into the scalp and leave it on for about ten minutes. (If you drape a towel around your head and lie on a slant board while the conditioner does its work, you will benefit doubly. See Chapter 13 for more information on slant boards.)

After ten minutes, thoroughly rinse the conditioner from your hair with warm water. Follow with your usual shampoo.

This high-protein, all-natural hair conditioner helps to dislodge debris clogging the tiny openings in the scalp, leaving them free for the passage of nutrients to the hair. It also enriches the hair, helping to make it stronger and more lustrous.

Camomile conditioner
Brew camomile as you would tea. 5ml (1 teaspoon) of the herb to 250ml (1 cup) of water is the usual proportion. Cool and

strain the brew. Dip your fingers into the liquid and thoroughly massage the entire scalp.

In addition to the foregoing, the following herbs, made into a 'tea', are excellent for stimulating the scalp and promoting hair growth. Apply the infusion by dipping the fingers into it and massaging it thoroughly into the scalp, as previously outlined.

- Henna leaves
- Marshmallow leaves
- Nettle
- Peach (kernels or buds)
- Pepper grass
- Rosemary
- Willow (leaves and bark).

These herbs may also be used in combination with boric acid (available from the drug store), thus:

Make a tea with the herb (already described) and add 15ml (a level tablespoon) of the boric acid. Stir well to mix. Massage the solution into the scalp.

Other conditioners
Other conditioners, already prepared for you and sold mainly at health food stores, contain ingredients such as sea kelp (a variety of seaweed), vitamins (including biotin) and apricot kernel oil to help to rebuild hair by replacing some lost protein and other nutrients. In kelp, for instance, many of the minerals and vitamins that are essential to healthy hair growth and regeneration, occur naturally.

Aloe vera
Aloe vera products are now gaining popularity for a variety of reasons, including the healing of cuts and sunburns and the relief of itching caused by some rashes.

These products are made from the aloe vera plant, the leaves of which produce a gel. The main constituents of the gel are two *aloins*, thought to contain healing properties.

Mexican Indians have long used aloe vera as a hairdressing. They rubbed the gelatinous juice oozing from the leaves of the plant into their hair and scalp. They left it on overnight and washed it off next day. No shampoo was necessary — the aloe produced its own rich lather. Their hair became beautifully shiny, full of body and was very manageable. The healing properties of the aloe were absorbed into the scalp in a matter of hours.

Jojoba

Jojoba (pronounced 'ho-ho-ba') products, made from the fruit of the jojoba plant, are also being recognized as a natural aid to healthy hair.

The jojoba is a desert shrub which is found chiefly in the southwestern United States, in Mexico, and in Israel. The fruit it bears produces an oil now being used in industry (as a lubricant) and for its food and medicinal value. The Papago, Yaqui and other Indians of the southwestern United States have long used the jojoba as food, medicine and a skin and hair tonic. They believed it to be an effective treatment for the hair and scalp.

A professor of dermatology at UCLA in California has been recommending jojoba products to his patients to help with skin and hair problems. In his clinical judgement, he remarked, jojoba appeared to be effective, and indeed his patients have reported that they seem to be getting results. The professor added that Mexicans have long been using jojoba — for about 400 years!

Apart from having lubricant and healing properties, jojoba also has a high protein content.

Cleansing

Shampooing

Although the occasional expert will suggest that washing the hair with shampoo is not advisable, the consensus of knowledgeable authorities on hair care is that the hair should be shampooed about twice a week, perhaps three times if the hair tends to be abnormally oily. Some even recommend a daily shampoo.

Those who argue against washing with hot water and soap or shampoo say that these remove the natural scalp oils, alter the condition of the scalp from acid to alkaline and cause dryness which promotes dandruff. They suggest that daily brushing of the hair will keep the scalp sufficiently clean, apart from a warm water hair wash as part of the shower bath. They concede, however, that since most people will not heed their advice and will continue to shampoo their hair, they should at least use an acid rinse to help to restore the scalp's acid mantle.

If you use a commercial shampoo such as those sold in drug stores, dilute it. Commercial shampoos tend to be too alkaline. Madison Avenue hairdresser Richard Stein has suggested mixing one part shampoo with seven parts water before using. Undiluted shampoos, he has emphasized, do not completely rinse out after each wash. He remarked that all commercial shampoos currently sold are far too concentrated to pour directly onto the hair and scalp. He further stated that barbers and hairdressers have always diluted shampoos before using them, but that this practice does not seem to have caught on in the home. So many scalp and hair problems, he observed, result from the film left by concentrated shampoos. People can reduce their hair loss by diluting their shampoo, as suggested.

Health food stores sell shampoos made with natural ingredients, and so formulated as to help to preserve the scalp's natural pH. An example of such a shampoo is that made from jojoba oil (see above). One man, who started losing hair from the age of twenty, noticed a new crop sprouting on the top of his head after he had been using a brand of jojoba shampoo for six months. Jojoba apparently helps to halt hair loss and energize hair growth naturally.

You will also find shampoos made with the various herbs already mentioned, as well as with sea kelp, vitamins and apricot kernel oil. Since these are all natural ingredients, they are compatible with the scalp and hair and help to enhance their health.

Protein-rich homemade shampoo
Try this high-protein shampoo which imparts body and sheen to the hair.

Beat together two eggs and 125ml (½ cup) lukewarm water. Use this mixture as you would ordinary shampoo, massaging it well into the scalp. Leave it on the hair for about fifteen minutes (if you drape a towel around your hair and lie on a slant board, you will be benefiting doubly).

After fifteen minutes, thoroughly rinse the hair with tepid water. *Do not* use very warm or hot water — you will end up with scrambled egg in your hair!

Shampoo technique

For best results, use a hose with a fine spray attachment, or your shower.

Thoroughly soak the hair and wet the scalp with warm water. Pour some shampoo into a palm and apply it to the hair and scalp, distributing it all over. Massage the entire scalp, using the manual massage technique described in Chapter 13, p.129-130.

Rinse the hair thoroughly with clean water. If absolutely necessary, shampoo again, working up to a generous lather and massaging the scalp carefully. Do not rush the massage — it is the most important part of your shampoo.

It is important, too, that the water does not strike the hair and scalp with great force. This strains and scatters the hair, thus promoting unnecessary tension and tangling.

Finish with an apple cider or herbal rinse (recipes below).

Post-shampoo rinses

Natural hair rinses help to ensure that all traces of shampoo have been removed from the hair and scalp. They also help to restore the scalp's natural acid mantle. Furthermore, acid rinses reduce the film of hard water salts that some shampoos deposit on the hair shafts. They impart lustre to the hair, making it truly a crowning glory.

Apple cider rinse

Mix together 15ml (1 tablespoon) apple cider vinegar and 250ml (1 cup) cool water. Pour over freshly shampooed hair. Rub in well.

Lemon rinse

Squeeze one large, fresh lemon. Strain the juice and mix it into 250ml (1 cup) cool water. Save the lemon rinds to steep in water to use as a final hair rinse.

Nettle rinse

Steep 15ml (1 tablespoon) nettle in 250ml (1 cup) of boiling water. Leave for half an hour. Strain and cool.

Nettles have been used for centuries for stimulating hair growth and preserving hair colour.

Camomile rinse
Make a 'tea', as for nettles, and use in the same way.

Three-herb rinse
Mix together 15ml (1 tablespoon) each camomile, raspberry leaves and rosemary.

Steep in about 550ml (1 pint) water, as if making a tea. Leave it for half an hour. Strain and cool. Pour into a bottle or jar and use as a post-shampoo rinse.

You may also use this mixture as a pre-shampoo conditioner.

Note: Rosemary is thought to have a good effect on the blood vessels. The oil or infused leaves are considered very beneficial for hair and scalp, and the oil is believed to stimulate the hair follicles and darken the hair.

Hairdrying

Ideally, you should gently towel-dry hair, comb it into style with a wide-toothed comb and let it dry naturally in the air.

When towel-drying, do not rub the hair. This increases the area subjected to undue friction, places unnecessary tension on the hair shafts and promotes damage.

It is best to pat the hair until the towel has absorbed most of the moisture.

Today's busy lifestyles, however, make this natural approach impractical for many persons. Furthermore, seasonal temperatures may not permit this method of hair drying in absolute comfort. And so we must resort to using the electric hairdryer more frequently than is perhaps best for the hair.

This being the case, electric hairdrying, sensibly managed, can be done without damage. The main thing to remember is not to subject the hair and scalp to high heat. Use a low or medium setting on the dryer, and do not over-dry the hair, especially if your hair already tends to be dry.

Do not hold the dryer too close to the hair or scalp (15cm or 6 inches is about right). It is best to diffuse rather than concentrate the heat on any one area at a time.

When the weather permits, do not routinely use your electric hairdryer. Towel-dry the hair and finish the drying process in the open air. The scalp and hair will be healthier for it.

Brushing and combing

These provide both cleansing and stimulation of the scalp for healthy, flourishing hair.

Daily brushing should be as important a part of your health care routine as eating, brushing your teeth and going to bed.

Brushing sweeps away from the scalp the dirt and dandruff and dead skin cells that accumulate there. These block the conduits for the passage of nutrients to the hair cells.

Although it is best to clear away built-up scalp wastes as promptly as possible so that the scalp pores can breathe, do not brush with a vengeance. The scalp is delicate tissue that requires respect.

British trichologist Philip Kingsley, however, does not advocate brushing. He recommends using a wide-toothed, saw-cut comb to remove foreign matter and stimulate scalp circulation. He considers the scalp living and fragile tissue to be protected and enhanced, and warns against beating it about every day with a brush or shocking it with too vigorous a massage!

Most other hair experts, however, suggest daily hairbrushing, provided that it is done correctly, as follows.

Hairbrushing technique
Stand with your feet wide apart. Bend forward at the hip joints to hang the head down (unless you have high blood pressure or other condition that prohibits this — *check with your doctor*).

Brush the hair from the nape of the neck, down the middle of the head, using long sweeping strokes. Brush down each side of the head. Slowly and carefully straighten up and brush the hair from the front of the head, across the top, down the back. Brush the hair at the sides of the head.

Do not rush the hairbrushing procedure. Spend between three and five minutes a day on it.

The right brush and comb
A good quality, natural bristle brush is the only brush worthy of those who truly care about their hair.

Nylon brushes tend to be too abrasive to the scalp. They can damage this delicate area and create sites for infection. Nylon combs, too, with their sharp teeth, are best left in the stores by those who want to maintain excellent hair.

A tortoiseshell comb is best. Choose one with blunt teeth, spaced well apart, and sufficiently rigid without being too hard on the scalp.

Natural bristle brushes and tortoiseshell combs are available in better health food stores and some beauty and barber supplies outlets.

Tip for cleaning combs and brushes
Save your lemon rinds, and steep them in water for washing combs and brushes.

Feeding the hair

The third vital key to vigorous hair growth and regeneration is food. Chapters 4 to 7 give details about nutrients that are essential to the life and renewal of the hair, the sources of these nutrients and the best ways of utilizing these substances. These chapters are worthy of review.

The herbal and other natural conditioners applied externally to the scalp are, to some extent, absorbed through minute openings. Although they must not be depended upon as the prime source of nourishment for the hair, they may be employed as useful aids to the overall nutrition of the hair. Whereas these conditioners are made from natural ingredients and give body and sheen and life to the hair, commercial counterparts tend to leave an unnecessary film that coats hair shafts and attracts dirt. Such products are to be shunned.

The following are additional ways in which to boost scalp and hair nutrition. Profit from them — your hair needs all the help it can get.

Recipes for improved hair growth

Healthy-hair beverages
To make these healthful beverages you will need an electric juice extractor, available from a large, reputable department store or a health food store. Some health magazines advertise juice extractors and tell where to obtain them. To get your money's worth, invest in a good quality juicer and use it daily.

Alfalfa drink

Throw into the juicer a generous handful of alfalfa sprouts (available at larger supermarkets or health food stores), half a dozen well-washed green lettuce leaves (do not use round lettuce) and a couple of scrubbed, chopped carrots. Extract the juice. Drink it immediately (storing causes vital nutrients to dissipate).

Alfalfa is very rich in chlorophyll, an element in plants comparable to haemoglobin (the colouring matter in red blood cells).

Because freshly pressed juices are easily assimilated, their nutritive substances pass into the bloodstream very readily and are conveyed to every body cell for its enrichment.

One man reported that, after taking the foregoing beverage for about three months, he grew a new crop of hair on his bald head.

High-mineral beverage

Loose leaf lettuce is high in the minerals iron and magnesium, both of which are important in red blood cell manufacture. For this reason alone, it is an excellent hair-restoring food.

Make a juice of lettuce, chopped carrots and celery. Let the lettuce be the predominant ingredient and remember to use only loose leaf lettuce. Drink the juice right away.

Green pepper cocktail

The key element in this cocktail is silicon which, you may recall, is a trace mineral that gives beautiful finishing touches to the scalp and hair.

Put a couple of medium-size, chopped-up green peppers (remove the seeds) into your juicer. Add two cut-up carrots and a small bunch of washed spinach. Extract the juice. Drink it immediately.

Cucumber beverage

Cucumber is diuretic — it helps to eliminate surplus fluid from the body, as well as waste matter; cucumber is cleansing — it helps to clear up undesirable scalp and skin conditions.

One health author suggests that, to improve hair growth, you should take about 550ml (1 pint) of freshly pressed natural vegetable juice a day. You can drink the juice at breakfast, between main meals and at bedtime.

For the cucumber beverage, put into your juicer a thinly peeled, medium-size, cut-up cucumber, two cut-up carrots and a small bunch of washed spinach or a few green lettuce leaves. Extract the juice and drink it straightaway.

Five-juice cocktail
Process the juice of these five vegetables combined: carrot, celery, parsley, spinach and watercress. Drink the cocktail right away.

This beverage is an excellent general tonic. Carrot and parsley are high in the 'skin' vitamin, A, and the green leaves are rich in iron.

In combination, these vegetables furnish several other minerals and vitamins needed for healthy blood — the life force of vibrant hair growth.

Blender beverages
Apart from the juice extractor, the single most important small electric appliance for anyone interested in keeping his or her hair and keeping it superbly healthy is an electric blender.

An electric blender is versatile — you can make anything from high-protein quick-bread mixes to 'instant' breakfast drinks in it, and for today's very busy person that is truly a boon.

Below are two recipes you will enjoy making and drinking, and which your scalp and hair will soak up gratefully.

Three-fruit shake
Remove the rind and seeds from a large chunk of watermelon. Cut up the fruit (yields about 500ml or 2 cups). Wash a medium-size or large, fresh peach. Remove the stone; leave or remove the skin. Wash six large, fresh strawberries. Remove the caps and stems.

Put all the fruit into the blender and blend until smooth. Drink (or eat) promptly.

High-protein milkshake
Into the blender put one cup of milk. Add 15ml (1 heaped tablespoon) powdered milk (instant or non-instant, preferably the latter, which is available at health food stores). Cover the blender. Blend well.

Uncover the blender. Add 5ml (1 teaspoon) unpasteurized honey and a flavouring of choice (such as a teaspoon of carob powder, also available at health food stores, for a 'chocolate' flavour; or a few drops of vanilla essence or grated nutmeg). Add the yolk of a fresh egg. Blend again, and drink.

Variations
You may incorporate your daily quota of nutritional yeast into the above basic milkshake. There are palatable varieties of this product on the market; some even dissolve instantly in liquid.

You may also stir instant nutritional yeast into a glass of unsweetened orange or pineapple juice, to boost your protein and vitamin B-complex intake.

Experiment, too, with adding cut-up fresh fruit in season to the basic milkshake. Possibilities are apple, apricot, banana, cantaloupe melon, cherries, peaches and pears (remember to remove stones).

13.
AIDS TO HEALTHIER HAIR GROWTH

In Chapter 9, I gave exercises to help your body counteract the effects of gravity. These upside-down and semi-reverse positions assist the blood circulation in getting to parts of the body it normally reaches only with some difficulty, namely, the scalp and hair. Without a sufficiently rich supply of blood with its hair-rejuvenating properties, the hair cells gradually languish and fail to renew themselves.

Not everyone, however, is able to do the headstand, for instance. For these persons, there is still hope. There are natural aids to fight the dragging-down, nutrient-robbing effects of gravity and to encourage an opulent supply of blood to the scalp.

The headstand stool

This aid simplifies the practice of the headstand. Its use is subject to the same cautions as those for the practice of the headstand itself.

The headstand stool consists essentially of a frame, with a support for the neck and upper back, onto which the practitioner can hold as he or she assumes the inverted position.

Several brands of headstand stool are available. Some can double as a footstool. They can be purchased at better health food stores and health supplies outlets. Some magazines, too, carry advertisements for these and other 'body inversion' products which, say the manufacturers, help you to get into position without any special strength, balance or agility.

The slant board

Available at some department stores, health food stores and medical supply houses, this board is perhaps one of the best investments you can make for the preservation and regeneration of your hair.

The slant board permits you to lie, in comfort, with the head down and the feet elevated. It allows the blood access to the tissues of the scalp with a facility not normally possible. This has a marvellously rejuvenating effect on all the organs, glands, blood vessels and other structures of the body, including sluggish hair cells which are then reactivated.

The slant board, in effect, provides a natural internal 'blood transfusion' that is without parallel, except by the headstand exercise held for several minutes daily.

How to make a slant board

You need a plank of board between 50 and 60cm (20 and 24 inches) wide, 180cm (6 feet) long and about 2cm (¾ inch) thick. If you are very tall, make the length of the board about 195cm (6½ feet).

You also need two sets (four in all) of folding legs between 27.5 and 50cm (15 and 20 inches) high, which you attach to the plank to make what is, in fact, a narrow bed or bench that doubles as a slant board when one set of legs is collapsed (Figure 21).

A foam mattress, about 7.5cm (3 inches) thick, and fabric long and wide enough to cover the plank, are useful.

A padded ironing board, too, may be used as a makeshift slant board. Prop the tapered end against something stable and lie with your head at the lower end.

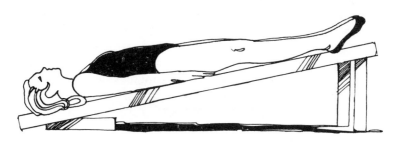

Figure 21 Using a slant board

To use the slant board

The same cautions for the practice of the shoulderstand exercise apply to the use of the slant board.

Lie on the board with your head at the lower end. Close your eyes. Breathe naturally. Relax as well as you can.

For best results, stay in this position for fifteen to twenty minutes. Use your slant board at least once a day, preferably twice.

In addition to being a hair-regenerator, the slant board is an excellent relaxation aid. Keep one at your work place, if possible. Use it whenever your energy flags or you experience tension build-up or you are exhausted. You will be amazed at its power of revival.

Helpful hint

While resting on the slant board, treat your scalp to a stimulating manual massage (see below).

Scalp massage

Hair scientists have offered persuasive evidence that a tight scalp prevents the hair from flourishing and contributes to abnormal hair loss. Chapter 10 presents some of these findings.

The overcontraction of muscles beneath the scalp causes excessive pressure on the tissues and the countless blood vessels located there. It greatly restricts the blood flow to the hair manufacturing plant (the papillae). Because of this impaired blood supply, the papillae fail to produce optimally — the cells they feed become impoverished and do not thrive. This may, and often does, lead to abnormal hair loss.

A tight scalp, then, is a potential threat to the health, growth and regeneration of the hair. A loose scalp permits the passage of hair-growing substances to the hair-manufacturing plant.

Stimulating the scalp tissues is, therefore, one of the critical elements in the maintenance of healthy hair growth. Some experts even consider that the first essential in the treatment of all hair problems is to *keep the scalp loose*. This loosening can be effected by the practice of scalp-stimulating exercises that reduce scalp tension and promote a plentiful supply of nutrient-rich blood to the hair cells. It can also be achieved effectively by regular and proper massage of the scalp.

Benefits of scalp massage

Massage of the scalp stimulates the blood circulation and improves it so that the hair cells, which are at the periphery, can be better nourished.

Massage helps the natural hormone secretions to become better absorbed so as to prevent drying of the scalp. It keeps the scalp supple and young.

Massage beneficially stimulates nerve endings in the scalp for the overall profit of the nervous system which is intimately related, functionally, to the glandular system. It relaxes the scalp muscles and reduces the tension that impairs blood circulation.

A final important benefit: massage effectively stimulates the flow of lymph to aid in the cleansing of the bloodstream. It is by means of lymph that nourishment and oxygen reach the various tissue cells, and dead cells and other debris are cleared away from the system. Lymph is vital to blood purification.

Manual massage

Some dermatologists caution that, unless you employ the correct massage technique, you may break off more hairs than you will invigorate. It is important not to tug at the hairs as you massage. It is the scalp that you must move, not the hair.

How to massage the scalp

1. Sit (or lie) comfortably where there is no impediment to free arm movement. (You may even stand to do your massage, if you have to.)
2. Slide the fingers of both hands through the hair at the back of the head (behind the ears). Press them firmly — but not unduly so — against the scalp. Maintain this gentle pressure throughout the massage.
3. Slightly tilt the head back to enhance the contact between scalp and fingers.
4. Move the fingers in a circular motion — one hand moves clockwise; the other counterclockwise. Do this several times. Sense the movement of the scalp, however slight. Rest.

5. Bring your head upright (adjust your head position, if you are lying down). Slide the fingers upward. Press them against a different area of the scalp. Repeat the circular massage movements, as before. Rest.
6. Repeat step 5 until the entire scalp, forehead and temples have been covered. Do not rush the procedure. Take at least five minutes, preferably eight to ten. It will be worthwhile.
7. Firmly massage the back of the neck by placing the fingers of each hand on the side of the cervical (neck) spine and rotating them several times.

Some experts suggest using the palms (the area near the thumb) rather than the fingertips, to carry out the massage action. Experiment, and choose the method you find more pleasurable and comfortable. But whichever you habitually use, be sure that it gives a gentle yet effective massage.

Helpful hints
Do this all-over scalp and neck massage when you shampoo your hair. Do it, too, when you lie on your slant board. Use it to revive you when fatigue sets in. It is a wonderful way to eliminate tension.

For best results, massage your scalp at least twice a day.

Vibrator massage
For effective, effortless massage, there are several brands of electric scalp vibrator on the market. Some have several attachments, one of which consists of projections especially suited to scalp massage.

It is important to read and understand how to operate the specific electric vibrator that you buy before actually using it. Philip Kingsley recommends the kind of vibrator that you strap on the back of the hand, but warns against the unit vibrator with the plastic brush or massage attachment. He considers this potentially harmful to hair and scalp because it can tangle the hair, break it, or injure the scalp tissue.

Whichever vibrator you decide to use, massage the scalp at least twice a day for best results. Use the same circular motion as in the manual massage until the entire scalp, forehead, temples and neck have been covered.

Helpful hints

Massage your scalp with your vibrator when you lie on your slant board. You will feel like a new person and your hair will thrive the better for it.

Practise the following exercise several times a day, during odd free moments, in traffic jams, while waiting for appointments — wherever you can do it unobtrusively.

Try to focus your attention on the scalp and to sense its movement as you do the exercise. If you rest your fingers lightly on the scalp near the forehead, it may help you to become aware of this. When you have become accustomed to the exercise and are finely tuned in to what is taking place, you need no longer use your fingers as a sensor.

The exercise

1. Sit or stand naturally erect. Breathe easily.
2. Inhale and raise your eyebrows, as if to push them toward the top of your head. This will wrinkle the forehead horizontally. Your eyes will open widely.
3. Hold this muscular contraction for a few seconds as you breathe normally.
4. Exhale and relax your forehead. Close your eyes (if possible). Visualize all tightness disappearing from scalp, forehead and eyes.
5. Open your eyes. Repeat steps 2 to 4 a few times. Repeat the exercise later in the day.

Two more simple exercises

The following two exercises, effective, easy to do and within reach of those unable to perform the headstand and shoulderstand, are excellent for encouraging a rich blood supply to the hair cells and for dissolving tension in the scalp, face and the rest of the body.

The dog stretch

Caution: If you have high blood pressure, *check with your doctor* before attempting this exercise.

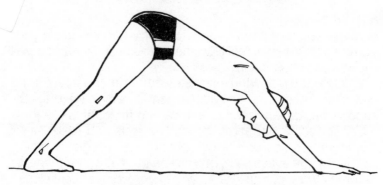

Figure 22 The Dog Stretch

1. Get on 'all fours' on your mat. Your thighs are roughly perpendicular to your torso; your arms somewhat sloping.
2. Tuck your toes in so they point forward.
3. Press on your palms and toes; raise your knees; straighten your legs and carefully push your heels downward (do not risk pulling the muscles at the back of the legs). Straighten your arms. Your hips are now raised and your head hangs downward (Figure 22).
4. Hold this position for a few seconds to begin with, breathing evenly. As you become accustomed to the posture, hold it for two to three minutes.

To come out of the position
Rock your body forward; lower your knees to the mat; relax the toes so that they point backward; sit on your heels and rest.

The mock headstand
This exercise sends a surge of fresh blood to the face, scalp and hair. It is also excellent for general relaxation.

Caution: If you have high blood pressure, do *check with your doctor* before trying this exercise.

How to do it

1. Sit on your heels.
2. Lean forward and lower your forehead to the mat, close to the knees.
3. Slowly raise your bottom from your heels — this will roll

the head until the top of it rests on the mat. Take care not to exert undue pressure on the skull. Hold on to your ankles or heels (Figure 23).

4. Hold this position for a few seconds only at first. *Do not hold your breath* — let it flow effortlessly. As you become used to this semi-inverted posture, maintain it for up to three minutes.

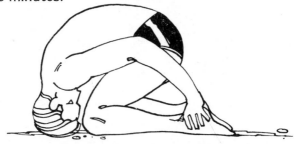

Figure 23   The Mock Headstand

To come out of the position
Very slowly ease yourself back toward your heels. Keep your head down for a few seconds before gradually sitting upright on your heels. Sit quietly for a few more seconds, breathing rhythmically, before getting up.

Watch your posture!

Proper carriage of the body is essential for maintaining the muscle tone of the whole system. When we indulge in faulty posture, be it when sitting or standing or walking, we cramp internal structures (such as blood vessels and glands) and their harmonious functioning is hindered.

For instance, if you habitually hang your head (which often accompanies rounded shoulders), you unwittingly restrict the blood flow in the neck arteries. These and their branches, you may recall, feed the scalp and hair. You therefore unconsciously detract from the optimal health of your hair.

One of the most common, albeit unsuspected, causes of general malaise or sluggishness is incorrect posture. It leads to a condition of *enteroptosis,* in which the stomach, intestines and sometimes the kidneys, liver and pelvic organs are dragged downward and remain in a position not compatible with optimum function.

Improper posture and carriage retard the blood circulation. They cause the blood in the abdomen to stagnate and this in turn contributes to constipation and to a general self-poisoning process.

We now know that it is by way of the bloodstream that every cell — not least of all the hair cells — is fed and activated. We also know that it is through the bloodstream that body wastes are eliminated. It is then not difficult to appreciate that faulty postures, which create unnatural pressure on internal structures, impede the blood circulation and interfere with its work of nourishing, regenerating and cleansing. Faulty posture, therefore, is detrimental to the health and thriving of the hair.

Statues and paintings and photographs of ancient Egyptian priests and pharaohs, of the Greeks, and of the Hindu deities are testimony that the ancients knew better than we the importance of the correct alignment of the spine. Apart from the dignity expressed by these elegant postures, a naturally erect vertebral (spinal) column is essential for the harmonious functioning of the nervous system. Innumerable nerves, you may remember, branch off the spinal column. If these become pinched through slouching and other unnatural positions, nervous system function is impaired. And since this system is intricately linked to the functioning of the endocrine glands and other vital structures, these are adversely affected also and yet another vicious circle is created.

Sit tall, stand tall and walk tall
To counteract the tendency to incorrect posture, then, a simple rule to remember is the one suggested by a doctor: sit tall, stand tall, walk tall — not, however, like a soldier with chest pushed out and back arched. This military attitude only exaggerates the natural arch at the small of the back (at waist level), and generates another set of problems (such as backache). Simply hold the body naturally erect. This almost automatically brings the spine into good alignment.

Relaxed standing
This is an exercise to bring you an awareness of what good posture looks and feels like. Practise it daily in front of a full-length mirror until it becomes second nature to you. Then apply its principles to sitting and walking.

1. Stand with the body weight equally distributed between the feet, which are close together. Relax your arms at your sides. Breathe regularly.
2. Hold the head up, but do not stick out the chin. The head is naturally poised.
3. Pull the shoulders down from the ears. Flatten the shoulderblades; relax the shoulders. To help, you may rotate your forearms so that the palms face forward.
4. Tilt your pelvis (hip region) so that there is no exaggerated curve at the small of the back. In other words, neither bottom nor chest should stick out.
5. Straighten, but not stiffen, your knees.
6. Think 'elegant'. Relax your jaws, face and the rest of your body. Hold this posture for about two minutes at first, perhaps working up to five minutes.

    You may turn sideways to the mirror to glance at yourself in profile.

Benefits
In this position, your thorax (chest cavity) is full rather than flattened. The diaphragm is high. The abdomen is at its longest so that all the structures it contains are freed from pressure by structures above. Muscular tensions are reduced.

The foregoing basic stance is regarded by physical education authorities as the most natural posture for standing. Apply its principles when you walk or sit.

GLOSSARY

Adrenal glands: ductless glands located on top of each kidney

Alopecia: deficiency of hair; baldness

Anagen: the growing stage of hair development

Androgen: a substance producing or stimulating male characteristics; a word used in general reference to any male hormone

Atherosclerosis: a hardening of blood vessels (arteries) with loss of elasticity due to a build-up of fatty material within them

Bulb (hair): the lower expanded portion of a hair 'root'

Catagen: the intermediate phase of the hair growth cycle, which occurs after the growth, or anagen, phase and before the resting, or telogen, phase

Cervical: pertaining to the neck

Cholesterol: a fat-like substance found in various places in the body (such as the blood, the brain) and in some foods

Dermatitis: inflammation of the skin

Dermatology: the science of the skin and its diseases

Diaphragm: the muscular dome-shaped partition separating the chest from the abdomen

Diuretic: an agent that increases the flow of urine

Endocrine gland: a ductless gland which produces an internal secretion (hormone)

Follicle (hair): the sheath in which a hair grows

Galea aponeurotica: a fibrous sheet of connective tissue covering the skull

Glabrous: smooth, bald

Haemoglobin: the colouring matter of red blood cells (it has a strong affinity for oxygen because of its iron content)

Hirsute: hairy

Hormone: the secretion of ductless (endocrine) glands, such as insulin which is secreted by the pancreas

Lymphatic system: the system including all structures involved in conveying lymph (a clear alkaline fluid) from the tissues to the bloodstream

Occipito-frontalis muscle: the muscle covering the skull; it runs from above the eyebrows to the back of the head and controls the movements of scalp and face (the *galea aponeurotica* is attached to this muscle)

Oestrogen: an endocrine secretion that stimulates the female generative organs to reproductive function; female sex hormone

Ovaries: a pair of glandular organs situated in the female pelvis; they produce hormones

Pancreas: a gland situated behind the stomach; it produces digestive fluids and hormones

Papilla (hair): a cone-shaped projection of inner scalp tissue, which fits into the hair bulb; it contains minute blood vessels through which the hair receives its nourishment

Parathyroid glands: four small endocrine glands, associated with each lobe of the thyroid gland, located in the neck

Periphery: the part away from the centre; the outer part or surface of the body

Pituitary gland: an endocrine gland suspended from the base of the brain; the hypophysis

Progesterone: a hormone that controls menstruation and pregnancy

'Root' (of hair): the part of the hair inside the follicle

Scalp: the external tissues covering the skull

Scurf: thin, dry scales or crusts on the scalp

Sebaceous glands: the oil-secreting glands of the skin

Seborrhoea: overactivity of the sebaceous glands

Seborrhoea capitis: seborrhoea of the scalp, popularly known as dandruff

Seborrhoea sicca: dry dandruff

Sebum: the oily secretion of the sebaceous glands

Shaft (of hair): the part of the hair projecting above the hair bulb

Subcutaneous: beneath the skin

Telogen: the resting stage of the hair growth cycle

Testicles: the two reproductive glands in the scrotum, which produce sperm and the male hormone, testosterone

Testosterone: an androgen, or male hormone, produced by the testicles. This hormone is also produced by the adrenal glands in both males and females

Thorax: chest

Thyroid gland: an endocrine gland located in front of the trachea (windpipe)

Trichologist: hair scientist

Urinalysis: chemical analysis of the urine

Vasodilator: an agent that causes dilation of blood vessels

BIBLIOGRAPHY

Airola, Paavo. *Stop Hair Loss*. Phoenix, Arizona: Health Plus Publishers, 1980

American Heart Association. *The American Heart Association Cookbook* (3rd ed.). New York: David McKay, 1979

Belsky, Marvin S. and Gross, Leonard. *How to Choose and Use Your Doctor*. New York: Arbor House, 1975

Benson, Herbert. *The Relaxation Response.* New York: William Morrow, 1975

Brauer, Earle W. *Your Skin and Your Hair.* New York: Macmillan, 1969

Brena, Steven F. *Yoga and Medicine.* Baltimore: Penguin Books Inc., 1973

Brooks, Stewart M. *Basic Science and The Human Body.* St Louis: C. V. Mosby, 1975

Burkitt, Denis. *Eat Right — To Stay Healthy and Enjoy Life More.* Scarborough, Canada: Prentice-Hall of Canada, 1979

Ceres. *Herbs for Healthy Hair.* Wellingborough, England: Thorsons Publishers, 1977

Cerney, J. V. *Handbook of Unusual and Unorthodox Healing Methods.* West Nyack, New York: Parker, 1976

Feinberg, Herbert S. *All About Hair.* New York: Simon and Schuster, 1979

Fryer, Lee, and Dickinson, Annette. *A Dictionary of Food Supplements.* New York: Mason/Charter, 1975

Kingsley, Philip. *The Complete Hair Book.* New York: Grosset and Dunlap, 1979 and England: Magnum Books, 1980

Kloss, Jethro. *Back to Eden.* New York: Beneficial Books, 1971 and England: Woodbridge Press, 1977

Lappé, Frances Moore. *Diet for a Small Planet,* revised edition. Ballantine Books, 1975

Lubowe, Irwin I. *New Hope for Your Hair.* New York: E. P. Dutton, 1960

Prevention Magazine (staff of). *The Complete Book of Vitamins.* Emmaus, PA: Rodale Press, 1977

Schoen, Linda Allen (ed.). *The AMA Book of Skin and Hair Care.* New York: J. B. Lippincott, 1976

Sternberg, Thomas. *More Than Skin Deep.* New York: Doubleday, 1970

Thomson, James C., and Thomson, C. Leslie. *Healthy Hair.* New York: Arc Books, 1969 and England: Thorsons Publishers, 1977

Wade, Carlson. *Natural Hormones: The Secret of Youthful Health.* West Nyack, NY: Parker, 1972

Williams, Roger J. *Nutrition Against Disease: Environmental Prevention.* New York: Pitman, 1971

INDEX